Among Me

The 4Gs of Healing:
A simple guide to navigate chronic illness.

BRANDIE SMITH

Printed in the United States of America

First Printing, 2018

Editor – Blake Gerrits

Designer – Rebecca Sheahan

ISBN-13:
978-1981809349

ISBN-10:
1981809341

www.amongme.com

CONTENTS

APPRECIATION

The source of all my strength, blessings, faith and hope is Jesus Christ.

My husband has been with me through every tear-filled day of my journey. No one makes my heart smile and lightens burdens like Ken. He is a strong man who lifts me up by his belief in me. Ken, you are my rock and the single best human being I have ever met. I am honored to be your wife and blessed to be with you every day, babe.

My son, Zack, is the reason I fight every day, and as his mother I would do anything to be there at his side. And not just be present, but enjoy running and playing with him in full health. Zack, I hope you see every day how deep my love is for you.

The scariest thing in my life thus far is not being able to care for my own son. My sister, Kimiyo, and mother-in-law, Theila, gave selflessly to put their lives on hold to care for my family. Your decisions to put your lives on hold and come were grand gestures of love that words are inadequate to communicate my level of gratitude for each of you.

Honor to the man who showed me how to sacrificially love like Jesus: my dad, Ray Williams. When I looked into my father's eyes, I saw the unconditional love that was the same yesterday, today and tomorrow.

There are so many others who have encouraged me in writing this book and I am grateful for you all: Bill and Kimiyo Williams, Barry Culbertson, Mike and Linda Smith, Reid and Andrea Smith, Scott Fowler, Mike Pousti, Angela Medina, Jordan Christy, Jamie Walton, Joanie Moes, Valerie McConnin, Ioanna Vouloumanou, Shanda Damphousse, Jan Biddick, Sally Winter, and the prayers by sweet Mona.

INTRODUCTION

Psalm 118:17 (NIV)
"I wil not die but live, and proclaim what the Lord has done."

When you go through a health crisis, everything is heightened: your mental, emotional, and physical capacities are taxed to their limits, and your nervous system is usually frayed. What you do next will largely determine the outcome of the crisis. Will you choose peace, prayer, and faith? Or will you choose fear, anxiety, and stress? Whether it's being diagnosed with an autoimmune or chronic disease, unexpectedly losing a loved one, or enduring a difficult family situation, we all encounter moments of crisis; the question is, what will you do with yours?

Among Me will tackle issues of health, mental stability, and emotional well-being all from a God-centered and Spirit-led angle. *Among Me* will show you how to come through your crisis stronger and healthier. Through the power of prayer and positive, Scripture-based thinking; diet; and exercise, God can, and will, turn any situation around for your good, if you'll let Him!

This book is a quick read. Someone who is not feeling well needs answers and a step-by-step easy plan, not a novel. This book is intended to give you a simple guide to follow without too much time investment.

Why I wrote this book.

Because God deserves the Glory. It's that simple. He has been a rock in my journey with chronic illness and everyday life. All the strength needed to fight is found in Him. Start there. If you need a relationship with Christ, please see a simple prayer in the back of this book to begin a relationship with Him.

This book contains my story. I am a mom, wife, and professional. I am also a child of the Most High God, just as you are. God orchestrated encouragement for writing this book through other Christian women He brought into my life with hormonal and autoimmune conditions. I realized that if three out of eight women in my Bible study had hormonal and autoimmune conditions, there must be millions of women who are battling this often-lonely journey that is full of fear and worry.

And all eight women had hardship in their life that they needed encouragement through or freedom from including toxic relationships, trust issues, abuse, or shame from their past. Life has different seasons and having the right tools enables you to have peace in the midst of a storm and experience deeper joy in the summer season of life.

My journey with POTS and chronic illness.

I was diagnosed with POTS (Postural Tachycardia Syndrome) in July of 2016. That was 1.5 years ago from today. I have gone from not being able to care for my 2-year-old son, drive myself, or walk outside my home (due to fatigue and lightheadedness) to working-out 70 minutes a day, off most medications, and enjoying a full home and professional life. My health condition was so bad, I had actually wrote my will and instructions to care for my son should I die. Physically, I felt my body was betraying me and I was barely holding on.

The healing process took all 4 Gs of Healing. While I am not "cured," my life is pretty much back to normal compared to what it was.

My heart is to help others suffering through the battle of chronic illness, eliminate fear, and enjoy the full lives God designed for us to have. A scripture that provides me strength is Psalm 118:17 (NIV):

"I will not die but live, and proclaim what the Lord has done."

So, here I am boldly proclaiming what the Lord has done! I will dive deeper into my story later in the book.

The 4 Gs of Healing have brought me through ten years of infertility, the death of my beloved father to pancreatic cancer, and physical healing from chronic illness. I want everyone who could be living fuller spiritual, mental, and physical lives to experience the same freedom I have found.

4 Gs of Healing

Because of my experience, a large portion of this book is focused on those with autoimmune and other chronic inflammation conditions. However, the 4 Gs of Healing apply universally to anyone who has or is experiencing a life crisis. For those without a chronic inflammation condition, the diet restrictions and medical portions of this book may not apply to you but may be useful for someone you love.

This book is a guide to walk you through the 4 Gs of Healing:

Glow: Taking care of our body is critical to healing. The body has an incredible ability to heal itself when operated and nourished correctly.

"Therefore, I urge you, brothers and sisters, in view of God's mercy, to offer your bodies as a living sacrifice, holy and pleasing to God--this is your true and proper worship." (Romans 12:1 NIV)

Gratitude: You must grow the health of your mind through the power of prayer and positive, Scripture-based thinking.

"...to be made new in the attitude of your minds." (Ephesians 4:23 NIV)

Give: We are built to need others *Among Me* in this journey – focus on how you can use your experience to help someone else.

"Do to others as you would have them do to you." (Luke 6:31 NIV)

Grace: He is *Among Me*. He is the center and the power of this book. God is always among us, strengthening us, healing us, and guiding us into a life of purpose.

"I can do all this through him who gives me strength."
(Philippians 4:13 NIV)

Memorize these verses and focus your mind on them when you face struggles. He will be among us.

Lord, thank you that you love each of us more than we can comprehend. I pray that each person reading this book would hear from you, experience guiding by the Holy Spirit in their healing journey spiritually, mentally, and physically, and would come to know you more through this time. Break off all chains that hold them back and beliefs (lies that they tell themselves or that have been spoken over them) that are not true. And fill them with the spirit of truth, faith, and courage in You. In Jesus's Name, Amen.

MY STORY

''''''''''''''''''''''''''''''

Before the diagnosis of POTS:

My health issues have been a long journey. Looking back, it all makes sense that I had an underlining chronic inflammation condition that went undiagnosed for about 13 years.

At first, I thought my conditions were gastrointestinal, hormonal, and food sensitivity to grains, dairy, and soy. I was partially right. These were legit symptoms I experienced; however, the root cause remained undetected.

Doctors noted that I had the estrogen and progesterone levels of a 90-year-old woman (I was 30 years old), and I would need to be on hormone supplements for estrogen and progesterone my whole life. I was without a menstrual cycle for years.

About a year later, I experienced hypothermia in Costa Rica due to dehydration. I was then diagnosed with hypothyroidism and diabetes insipidus.

Diabetes insipidus is an uncommon disorder that causes an imbalance of water in the body. This imbalance leads to intense thirst even after drinking fluids (polydipsia), and excretion of large amounts of urine (polyuria). An MRI was also performed due to diabetes insipidus being so rare and attempting to find if there was a root cause. A small lesion measuring 3.7 mm was found on the pituitary gland. This could result in a reduction of hormones being released in my body.

At first, my hypothyroidism dosage of Synthroid was low (25 mcg/day) and I was put on desmopressin for diabetes insipidus to help me retain water. However, the Synthroid dosage grew over the years to be at 160 mcg/day.

Meanwhile, the gastrointestinal bloating, constipation, and food sensitiveness remained. I rotated through different treatments in hope of a cure including many common treatments such as L-glutamine, apple cider vinegar, psyllium husks, acupuncture, TUMS, and heartburn over-the-counter medications. Most of these alleviated some of the symptoms but the symptoms would return.

For the most part, I was able to continue my normal life and just learned how to adjust life to get through the daily bloating and food sensitivities However, there were many events that I didn't attend or left early because I simply felt bloated, lightheaded, or tired.

My heart vitals on all tests and from multiple visits to different cardiologist were extremely healthy. My heart was compared to an elite athlete's (average heart rate of 40 and blood pressure about 100/50); yet, I was in the ER at least once a year due to a racing heart and inability to breath or a heart rate so slow I thought I would fade out into a black cloud.

Through those 13 years, I lost count of how many doctors I visited. From a colonoscopy to blood work to ER visits, my counsel of doctors included endocrinologists, gastroenterologist, urologist, cardiologists, and ER care medics.

I must stop here to thank God and my husband. Every time I had an episode whether it was daily stomach bloating or an ER visit, I had peace. First, the peace that came from God. I experienced His peace that surpasses all (including my) understanding of the moment. And second, the peace my compassionate husband, Ken, gave to me.

The day when everything changed.

I lost my father in January 2016 to a 2-year battle with pancreatic cancer. This was two years filled with many beautiful life discussions with my beloved father as well as continuous stress watching someone I love suffer through one of the worst battles this planet has to offer the human race. I mention this here because my father's battle against cancer was my personal battle against cancer. I was determined to save him and trying to find a solution put me in the ER a couple of times. I was burning the midnight oil researching doctors and clinical research studies. I put the weight on my shoulders not to let down the man who never let me down. Letting go of him was intensely hard, but not as hard as watching the strongest man I ever knew suffer physically and emotionally every day.

In July 2016, my son got a nasty chest cold and shortly following, so did momma and daddy. My son, Zack, and husband, Ken, recovered quickly from the chest cold. However, within a matter of days, mine got worse. The chest cold symptoms seemed to fade after a few days, but were replaced by their ninja fighting cousins that brought more intense symptoms.

At first, I thought I must have a lung infection, like pneumonia, because of the inability to walk without physical exhaustion. I have never been so physically worn out in my life. Just walking up my stairs required me to physically lie down and recuperate. The fatigue got worse over the next couple of days. In fact, if I stood for a few minutes, I would feel faint and my heart would either have a dull, stabbing pain or start to race. Sometimes I would feel my breath quickening. It was difficult to stay vertical long enough to shower.

I went to the ER where they ran a series of tests on my chest, heart, and blood. All were fine - so frustrating.

Out of fear of not being able to care for my young son, I called every physician who may have a remote chance of knowing what was wrong with me. I was motivated to solve whatever was wrong with me, so I could care for my son.

My amazing mother-in-law, Theila, and sister, Kimiyo, came to care for Zack while I was at my worst, but I knew they needed to return home and I needed answers.

By the grace of God, I was diagnosed within 2 weeks (unheard of for those with autoimmune or chronic inflammation conditions) with Postural Orthostatic Tachycardia Syndrome ("POTS"), but the road to get a diagnosis was rough. The first cardiologist and endocrinologist misdiagnosed me with iron anemia. I got iron toxicity and that complicated matters. I wore a heart monitor for a week and was in two different doctor offices each day searching for an answer. My devoted family was driving me to and from doctor offices while also caring for my son. One day, I had to go the ER due to a racing pulse and inability to stand, got stabilized, and headed to my already scheduled doctor's visits to find a cure. On this particular day, my husband got in a car fender-bender with my son on the way to get me from the ER. The stress level was high. I was desperate.

Some doctors were not useful. After telling one neurologist that I thought I might have POTS and would like to be tested, he said I just seemed stressed and suggested seeing a psychologist. Yes, I was stressed - I went from running six miles a day to being unable to care for my son or stand long enough to shower!

Within two weeks, I was in the ER twice and had appointments with two cardiologists, three endocrinologists, an internal medicine doctor, two primary care doctors, a pulmonologist, a rheumatologist, an urologist, and two neurologists.

I had to demand a tilt test and heart monitor, even though my cardiologist thought I didn't need one. A tilt test is the best way to determine if one has POTS. It is important to push and be your own advocate. You are the only one who lives with your symptoms every day, and you know them best.

Here are the symptoms I had leading up to this diagnosis: racing heart, heart palpitations, chest pain (dull), tightness in chest, shortness of breath, pounding heart, chills, pale skin, nausea, headache, lightheadedness, fatigue, muscle soreness, pain in bones, jittery, twitching eyes, tingling in hands, and swollen lymphoid under chin upon waking up.

This began my intense journey for healing. I was too young to live in fear every day.

A year later, I discovered I have an autoimmune condition. It is unclear if the autoimmune triggered POTS or if POTS triggered the autoimmune condition. However, it was clear that I would need to be intentional in treating the complex web of chronic conditions my body was fighting: hormonal, diabetes insipidus, POTS, and autoimmune.

In my journey, healing encompassed honoring the way God created me in four distinct areas:

Glow: God created the body with an incredible ability to heal itself, given the right nutrients and by the removal of inflammation from the body.

Gratitude: I had to believe God would heal me and remove all the doubts that attempted to plague my mind. Your thoughts will shape your behaviors, which will shape your actions. I spoke truth (scripture) over my circumstance. It gave me courage and protection in my darkest hours.

Give: God allows situations in our lives, so we can use those to bless others. I started a blog to share my experiences with others who are suffering from chronic conditions.

Grace: Prayer (both privately and with your church body). I prayed God would heal me quickly. Healing has been an on-going journey, and He used this situation to heal my soul first. His perspective on healing is far greater than ours.

Today, I am off of all medications (except desmopressin for diabetes insipidus), including estrogen and thyroid hormones with test results in normal ranges.

I am still in a state of healing, but my severe chronic symptoms are in remission and are not preventing me from living and enjoying a full life every day.

My passion is to share my journey as I strive for better and better health. And to learn from all of you as we heal together and celebrate new levels of physical, mental, and spiritual health.

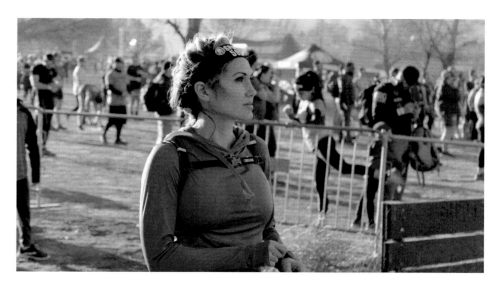

Competing in an extreme sports event in January 2018. This was a personal goal of mine when I got sick - to get my life back and participate in a physically competitive event.

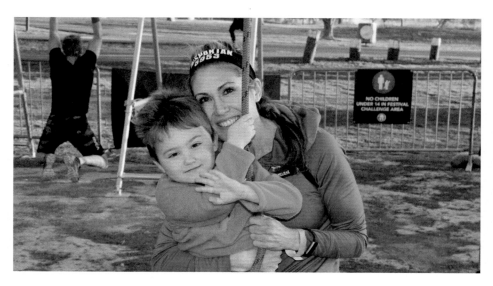

One of my biggest fans, Zack, preparing to cheer on his momma.

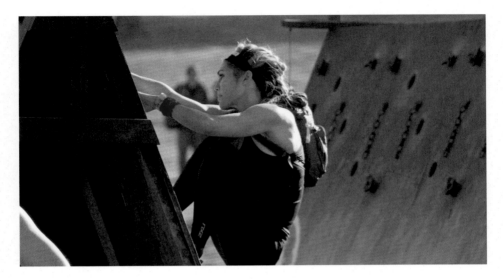

It was a tough event and the physical ability to participate was a blessing of which I enjoyed every minute.

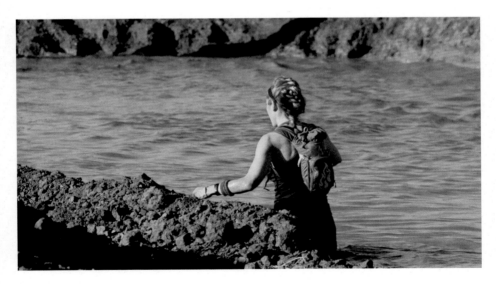

A personal come-back milestone in my journey of healing.

INFORMATION

James 1:5 (NIV)
"If any of you lacks wisdom, you should ask God, who gives generously to all without finding fault, and it will be given to you."

′ ′

What is an autoimmune condition?

Antibodies are proteins created by your own immune system to protect you from pathogens, like bacteria and viruses. The human immune system has the ability to create billions of different antibodies[1], each one meant to protect us from a different pathogen. Unfortunately, sometimes the antibody formation process goes awry, and the antibodies created by your immune system can turn against your own cells. These trouble-making antibodies are called autoantibodies. Autoantibodies can attack, damage, or interfere with the functioning of healthy tissues and cells in your body.

The American Autoimmune Related Diseases Association (AARDA) estimates that more than 50 million Americans[3] (roughly 1 in 6) suffer from autoimmune diseases, 75% of which are women[3]. Autoimmune is one of the top ten causes of death in women under the age of 65, the second highest cause of chronic illness, and the top cause of morbidity in women in the United States and around the world.[4]

Autoimmune is one of the most widespread epidemics with more than 100 autoimmune diseases[3]. According to the AARDA (in the US), more than $100 billion[3] is spent annually on the conventional treatment of this condition.

While the number of people with this condition is increasing, it remains inadequately understood. Autoimmune may include any organ or system in your body including hormonal, connective, nerve, muscle tissue, joint, skin, digestive, heart, and blood circulation.

It seems that the conditions people experience with autoimmune are vastly different at times; however, the commonality of an immune system attacking itself unites them all together. It is this diversity of symptoms that often makes getting quick and proper treatment difficult because the organs or systems in which these symptoms manifest spread the care across multiple medical disciplines.

Here are some of the symptoms that autoimmune patients have reported:
- Acid reflux
- Acne
- ADD/ADHD
- Allergies
- Alzheimer's
- Anxiety
- Arthritis
- Asthma

- B12 deficiency
- Blood clots
- Brain fog (difficulty focusing thoughts)
- Cardiovascular disease
- Depression
- Digestive issues (gas, bloating, indigestion, constipation, diarrhea)
- Dry eyes
- Eczema
- Fatigue
- Fibrocystic breasts
- Gallstones
- Hair loss
- Headaches
- Infertility
- Joint pain
- Muscle pain
- Obesity or excess weight (especially around middle section)
- Pancreatitis
- Sleep problems
- Swollen, reddened or painful joints
- Uterine fibroids

One of the most useful resources I've read about autoimmune and its root cause, triggers, and treatments is *The Autoimmune Solution* by Amy Myers, M.D.[6]

There are multiple medication options for treating autoimmune symptoms and these are well covered in another great resource: *The Autoimmune Wellness Handbook* by Mickey Trescott and Angie Alt[5]. Medication options will vary based on the type of autoimmune condition you have. You should consult with your medical team to determine the best treatment plan for you.

And as you heal your body with the tools you'll learn in this book as well as the recommended resources herein, the aim is that you'll be able to reduce the amount of medication you are on (in partnership with your medical team) and enjoy a fuller life. The goal is to address the root cause of current autoimmune condition and prevent flares and additional autoimmune conditions in the future. Approximately 25% of those with autoimmune disease will develop additional autoimmune diseases.[5]

Lifestyle Changes that Don't Require Medication:

1. *Lifestyle Changes.* Acute, short-term stress is useful in some circumstances but not as a lifestyle. Chronic stress is well understood to be a contributing trigger for autoimmune conditions and can cause flares because of its impact on the hormonal system. [6]

   In my case, a perfect storm of my father's battle and death from pancreatic cancer combined with leaky gut, an underlying autoimmune sensitivity, a nasty viral chest cold, and lack of nutrients (I was a "junkatarian" - ate vegetables, no meat, a lot of protein bars, and salty snacks with little nutritional value) triggered POTS.

   If you are like me, you may see stress as a challenge. Something you hold on your shoulders because others need you to be the strong one, or you feel you are the most equipped to carry the burden. Maybe feelings of guilt or shame cause you to take on more than you should. Life situations that cause an imbalance of emotional and hormonal energy need to be examined so we can determine what we have control over, what is ours to carry, and what we need to let go of and let God carry.

2. *Positive and Scripture-based Thoughts:*

If you spend just a few minutes researching your symptoms on the Internet, you'll find evidence that you will be on medication for the rest of your life, won't be able to enjoy a full life, and may even die. Our attitudes and actions follow our thoughts, which are moldable based on what we allow into our mind.

When I was diagnosed with POTS, I was provided zero insight on how such a condition would affect my life. This led me to the Internet to research whether I would get better and resume my life. A few hours later I was in tears and scared. I envisioned my son growing up without a mom. Who would ever love him as much as I would?

Thankfully, at the same time, a friend, Jan Biddick, emailed me an introduction to her sister, Sally Winter, whose daughter has POTS. I immediately called her and she filled me with such hope. She assured me that life would be normal again and that I was not going to die. This is how quickly negative input can affect our outlook and how quickly it can provide hope. From that day forward, I set my mind to doing that which Sally assured me was possible -getting my life back!

Knowledge is useful to empower you to address the root cause of your condition and find additional methods for coping and healing; however, look for sources of truth that saturate your mind with positive expectations and treatments rather than blogs filled of stories about how terrible the symptoms can be. Explain to caring friends who inquire about "how you're feeling" that you would rather not focus on the symptoms but rather enjoy the life you have. That this decision helps you heal by keeping your mind focused on the life you have in front of you.

You may have a chronic condition. It may not be curable. *But*, the symptoms can be manageable with the 4 Gs of Healing. You can still live a full life. And even during the tougher moments, you can experience the peace of the Lord that transcends all understanding.

3. *Exercise.* There are plenty of good reasons to work out beyond improvement of physical appearance. Exercise helps prevent disease, strengthens bones, improves mental health, may help you sleep better,[7] and enables the flow of the lymphatic system[8], which provides the body needed detoxification and immune function.

    However, there is a balance of movement without over exercising for those with autoimmune conditions. Too much exercise may have damaging effects on the immune system. Some signs of over exertion may include severe fatigue, immune system deficits, mood disturbance, physical complaints, sleep difficulties, and reduced appetite.[9]

I am dedicated to working out. I believe research outlining its benefits and personally feel it is critical in healing. At the beginning it is tough and starting with walking or a horizontal bike is a great first start.

For those of you who are just starting to work out, there is a weekly step-by-step guide at the end of the book in the 6-Week 4 Gs of Healing Plan. For individuals who have been working out and could handle a more challenging plan, there is a workout plan at www.amongme.com/resources.

4. *Diet.* This is where healing starts. Diet is so important that it is covered in great detail in the Glow section of this book. If you currently have an autoimmune condition, then you most likely have leaky gut (unless you've been treated for it).[6]

Conditions/symptoms that can signal leaky gut:[10]
- arthritis
- allergies
- depression
- eczema
- hives
- psoriasis
- chronic fatigue syndrome or fibromyalgia

Conditions/symptoms likely with leaky gut:[10]
- pain in multiple joints
- a chronic skin condition
- chronic diarrhea or abdominal pain

- chronic fatigue
- chronic depression
- malaise
- a feeling of being infected for which doctors aren't able to identify a cause.

I felt faint and nauseas every day until I used the elimination diet to remove all potential inflammatory foods from my diet, allowing my gut to heal, and then systematically reintroduce foods into my diet - testing which ones caused an adverse reaction in my body. Imagine my surprise when I found out the egg whites, which I ate two to three times a day, where the cause of the nausea!

In the Glow section of this book, you'll learn how to provide your body the nutrients it needs for recovery and healing. And just as important, in the 6-Week 4 Gs of Healing Plan, there is a week-by-week guide to show you how to test which foods might be causing inflammation in your body and undesirable symptoms. The goal is inflammation removal!

What is POTS?

Postural orthostatic tachycardia syndrome (POTS) is a form of dysautonomia that is estimated to impact between 1,000,000 and 3,000,000 Americans.[11]

There is some discussion in the medical community that POTS itself may be considered an autoimmune disorder; however, currently there is not sufficient evidence to qualify it as one completely. This is partially due to the fact that POTS is a relatively new diagnosis and there are not many proven treatments for this condition as the treatment for each person varies. However, it seems that many people diagnosed with POTS have an underlying autoimmune condition and the Leaky Gut treatment for autoimmune is also effective for POTS.

Here are some of the symptoms POTs patients have reported:[12]

- Abdominal pain
- Abnormal sweating
- Bladder Dysfunction
- Brain Fog (difficulty focusing thoughts)
- Chest Pains
- Chronic Pain
- Dizziness
- Faintness
- Fatigue
- Headaches
- Heart Palpitations
- Insomnia
- Nausea
- Shortness of Breath
- Sweating Abnormalities
- Tremors
- Weakness

The most useful site I've found is the *POTS Syndrome: Ultimate Guide* at http://myheart.net/pots-syndrome/.

There are medication options for treating POTS symptoms. I won't cover those in this book as they are already well covered in the POTS syndrome guide above. And hopefully, with the guidance of your medical team, you'll be able to reduce the amount of medications you require, as you get healthier through the tools you'll learn in this book.

There are a great number of patients, including myself, that have experienced symptom relief by natural, homeopathic, and lifestyle changes. In some cases, it may be useful to do both. You'll need to consult with your medical professional to navigate the right combination for you.

My personal journey saw some immediate relief by adding 8+ grams a day of salt to my diet under the care of a medical professional which helped manage some of the POTS symptoms. However, deeper physical and spiritual healing for me came through the 4 Gs of Healing over a year and a half. Now, it's rare to have to have even a couple of hours a month where I am not able to do what I want to do. Compared to where I came from, physically that feels like a gift and a miracle to me. I am so grateful.

Lifestyle Changes that Don't Require Medication:

1. *Positive and Scripture-based Thoughts*: "Above all else, guard your heart, for everything you do flows from it." *Proverbs 4:23 (NIV)*

   The Word is active and intended for our use every day in all circumstances. Our prayers and thoughts do not have creative power as such is the job of the God alone. Only God can heal. However, our prayers and thought-life do have the power of agreement, and we can stand in agreement with the truths of God's Word for our source of strength, peace, and hope. Focus on scriptures and scripture-based meditations throughout your day that breathe life into your soul.

God created our mind and understands how to operate it for optimal health. Everything you do is first a physical thought in your brain. You think, and then you act. You act and new memories build on and change the original thought. This dynamic relationship continues between thoughts and actions.[13] Hence if your thinking is positive, then your actions and communications are positive. The same is true if your thinking is toxic. Your thought-life will eventually be reflected in your outward communication, actions, and physical health.

2. *Lifestyle Changes.* Often POTS symptoms are worse in the morning. It may be helpful to have a more relaxed schedule in the morning. It is also important to get eight hours of sleep to enable your body to heal. If you have more severe symptoms in the morning, I have found it helpful when your first symptom hits in the morning, to have a natural electrolyte delight (recipe in the Glow section of this book). I usually feel better within a few minutes.

Each POTS patient is different. I have found it useful to schedule shorter outings so that I don't spend five hours at the beach. Rather, I go for two hours and then come back to home base where there is water, salt, food, and a place to rest if needed. Plan to have enough small snacks with you that, if needed, you could have eight ounces of water and salt every two hours if needed. If you don't need them, great! If you do, you'll be prepared and won't carry the mental stress of not having the resources you need if you do.

Track what times in the day your symptoms are more intense or frequent. Try to plan events that are more stressful or time sensitive for you outside of those time periods, if possible.

3. *Exercise.* Just like with autoimmune and other chronic inflammation conditions, exercise has been proven in all cases to improve the quality of physical and mental life, even for those suffering from pain and fatigue. Exercise can increase cardiac performance and muscle mass. Such increase will improve the body's natural ability to cope with long-term chronic conditions and stress.[7]

Of course, finding the right level of intensity and type of exercise that is right for you is equally as important. A good place to start is the week-by-week exercise progression plan in the 6-Week 4 Gs of Healing Plan found at the end of this book.

Some of you are reading this section and rolling your eyes because you can't even get out of bed. I understand, I've been there. Keep doing all that you can to reduce inflammation in your body, soul, and mind. It may be just baby steps for you right now. Do what you can do as your body allows...and just keep your eyes focused on God as you walk forward in faith. He still sees you. You are not alone. He is with you. Be still and lean on Him to fight for you. Use this down time to focus on strengthening your spirit (Grace) and mental health (Gratitude) while you wait upon the Lord for results.

4. *Diet.* For those with POTS, alcohol, and energy drinks should be avoided. You may be able to handle a small amount of caffeine, but many have found it useful to avoid caffeine altogether as it may trigger an episode.[14] Following the leaky gut diet has also been shown to help POTS patients (except don't follow the diet's low salt recommendation).

I found the most relief by following the autoimmune diet or AIP diet (except the reduction of sodium). You can Google these diets to find clear guidelines on following the criteria for the diet. Here are a few good resources:

- Amy Meyers M.D.'s book named *The Autoimmune Solution: Prevent and Reverse the Full Spectrum of Inflammatory Symptoms and Diseases.*
- Sarah Ballantyne PhD. www.thepaleomom.com
- Mickey Trescott NTP and Angie Alt, NTC, CHC, book named *Autoimmune Wellness Handbook: A DIY Guide to living well with chronic illness.*

These resources outline the process for eliminating foods that cause inflammation and contains easy-to-follow recipes. Diet is so important that it is covered in more detail in this chapter. Of course your integrated or functional medical provider would be the first place to consult before starting any new diet program.

5. *Fluid Intake.* Those with POTS should have 2+ liters of water a day. When experiencing lightheadedness or dizziness, it is recommended to drink 2 glasses of water over several minutes to help raise blood pressure and improve symptoms.[14] Personally, I've found that sometimes this needs to be done in combination with salt.

6. *Increase Salt.* POTS patience may experience symptom relief by taking up to eight grams of salt throughout the day with plenty of water as noted above.[14] Personally, I have found that I felt better on Himalayan Pink salt or Redmond Real Salt rather than the table salt tablets provided by the pharmacy. Therefore, I purchase my own salt from Costco and fill capsules myself. You can purchase capsules and a capsule holder with tamper on Amazon and make your own pills.

   For the first year, I was taking 12+ grams of salt a day. When I started to see the results of following the 4 Gs of Healing, I was able to drop my salt intake from 12+ grams a day to about six to eight grams a day (and I take no other medications outside of the desmopressin at night for diabetes insipidus to retain water) and supplements to support my immune system and overall health.

7. *Compression Devices.* Compression stockings, socks, and workout leggings help prevent blood from pooling in your feet and lower legs. The most effective compression garments will be at least 33 mmHg.

   Personally, I have found compression stockings that are full length to the waist are most effective; however, they are not always practical and stylish. I always wear them when flying and it helps.

When I am working out, I wear 2XU leggings (www.2xu.com) with compressions socks under my leggings. This is an essential for me to reduce symptoms from blood pressure drop after a good cardio workout. However, most health insurance companies won't cover leggings from 2XU. For daily wear compression stockings and socks, JUZO is a good brand and may be covered by your insurance. Given that compression stockings can be $100- $120, checking with your health insurance for approved dealers is wise.

Treatments for all chronic inflammation:

Autoimmune and POTS are considered (in most cases) to be chronic and not curable. Nevertheless, a full life is possible by reducing inflammation and toxins, and making certain lifestyle changes.

Whether you have an autoimmune condition, POTS, depression, GI issues, or another chronic condition, there are common mental, spiritual, physical, and dietary changes that you can make to improve your quality of life today.

Let's look at the common themes for healing inflammation in the spirit, mind and body.

<u>Glow:</u>

1. *Heal infections.* Certain infections can trigger an autoimmune condition or cause a flare for those with an autoimmune. Have your doctor run blood tests to determine if you have one of these common viruses in the herpes family: herpes simplex and Epstein-Barr.

Approximately 90% of Americans have antibodies to one or both of the herpes simplex viruses.[15] Herpes is not curable.[16] Sometimes, it is dormant and you may not notice its symptoms.[6]

Epstein-Barr is in the herpes family (along with genital herpes, cold sores, chicken pox, and shingles) and is a virus you acquire when you have mononucleosis (mono). Approximately 95% of adults in the United States have been affected with Epstein-Barr by the age of 35 to 40.[17] You can be exposed to Epstein-Barr and never have any symptoms. Once you've obtained the virus, you'll always have it.[6]

Active herpes and Epstein-Barr can be treated with antiviral medications, which can be prescribed by your medical professional. In her book, *The Autoimmune Solution: Prevent and Reverse the Full Spectrum of Inflammatory Symptoms and Disease*, Amy Myers, M.D. recommends the use of supplements in her healing protocol including L-Lysine, Lauricidin, and Humic Acid.

2. *Heal the gut.* 70-80% of the immune system is in your intestinal tract.[18] So common sense would tell us that in order to heal our immune system, we must heal our gut. This includes removing all gluten – a protein found in wheat, rye, barley, and many other grains contributes to gut inflammation and may cause leaky gut or an autoimmune condition.

Leaky gut (intestinal permeability) is a condition that happens as a result of intestinal tight junction malfunction. "Tight junctions" are the gateways between your intestines and what is passed into your blood stream. When this happens, undesirable things, such as gluten, bad bacteria, undigested food particles, and toxic waste, can pass through to your bloodstream causing an immune response.[19]

When this permeability of the intestines happens, it causes inflammation throughout your body and has been linked to:

- Allergies
- Asthma
- Autism
- Autoimmune disease
- Eczema and psoriasis
- Inflammatory bowel disease
- Rheumatoid arthritis
- Systemic inflammatory response syndrome
- Type 1 diabetes

Symptoms of leaky gut include:

- Food sensitivities: Due to the intestinal permeability and toxins entering the blood steam, the immune system produces various antibodies that attack antigens in certain foods, especially gluten and dairy.[20] Yet, those antibodies may also attack proteins in foods that look similar to those in gluten and dairy such as corn, oats, and rice.[21] Therefore, it is important to follow a proper elimination diet to determine which foods are causing inflammation in your body. We'll explore week-by-week how to integrate this diet strategy into your life in the 6-Week 4 Gs of Healing Plan at the end of this book.

- <u>Malabsorption of key vitamins and minerals:</u>   Various nutritional deficiencies are a result of leaky gut, including vitamin B12, zinc, and iron.[19] It is recommended that people with leaky gut take a whole food based multi-vitamin, live probiotic, L-Glutamine, licorice root (DGL), and digestive enzymes to help get the nutritional value needed from food.[19] You may also find that you need to take supplements for vitamins and minerals you are deficient in. You should schedule blood work with a functional doctor to identify nutritional deficiencies.

- <u>You have an autoimmune disease or high antibody markers:</u> Diet, toxins, medications, and lifestyle are all contributors to leaky gut. Leaky gut is an essential precondition to developing an autoimmune condition. If you have an autoimmune condition, likely you have leaky gut, unless it has been treated, and it would be wise to discuss with your functional medicine doctor.

    If you live in a location that does not have a functional medicine doctor, there are functional or integrated medicine professionals that take clients online now.

- <u>Thyroid problems:</u> Hashimoto's disease, an autoimmune condition that leaky gut may directly affect, is associated with hypothyroidism, fatigue, depression, weight gain, and decreased metabolism.[20]

- Inflammatory skin conditions: Intestinal permeability can be the root cause of a variety of skin conditions including acne and eczema. Generally, creams and drugs with harmful side affects are prescribed for these skin conditions that could be treated by healing the gut.[20]

3. *Get Moving.* Whether you have a chronic illness, unexpectedly lost a loved one, or enduring a difficult family situation, your body is under stress and toxins are building up in your system. Your lymphatic system has no pump and exercise is needed to remove toxins from your body.[8] Get moving and you'll feel better. If you've been sedentary before you began this program, start slow.

Gratitude:

1. *Think on positive, scripture-based thoughts and prayers.* "Finally, brothers and sisters, whatever is true, whatever is noble, whatever is right, whatever is pure, whatever is lovely, whatever is admirable - if anything is excellent or praiseworthy -think about such things" (*Philippians 4:8*). Make a decision to set your mind and keep it set on positive expectations. Consider flares as momentary; remember that you have overcome them before. They are not here to stay but to visit on your journey toward healing. Each flare gives you valuable knowledge on how to adjust the nutrients your body needs and remove agents of inflammation. This is a journey traveled one milestone at a time.

<u>Grace:</u>

1. Heal soul infections. Stress can spark a chronic condition or cause a flare up for those who already have an illness. Lightening the continual load of stress on the immune system will be vital in reversing symptoms. God knew we would face trials in this life, and He gave us the Word for comfort, peace, and healing. Therefore, be intentional and meditate on His word for daily strength and hope. It is hard to let go of certain matters; otherwise, you would have already done it. You must intentionally choose faith, and let the outcome be in God's hands.

If there is a known area of relationship discord where forgiveness needs to be offered or an area of your life that is not aligned with your core spiritual values, it will be a source of deep stress within your soul. Do not be fooled, ignoring these issues is not healthy. There is a physical and mental tax you will pay for issues avoided. Your body can't handle this amount of stress. Face each challenge with 100% grace combined with 100% truth at the same time. You may not agree, but we can disagree agreeably.

"If it is possible, as far as it depends on you, live at peace with everyone" (Romans 12:18 NIV).

Please be clear that I am not suggesting you are ill due to a discord in relationships or stress from work, home, or another situation alone. However, if there is a known or unknown stressor (rooted by being out of alignment with your deepest spiritual convictions), it is likely affecting your physical health, and is worth exploring with the Holy

Spirit, so you can experience total spirit, mind, and body freedom and healing.

Give:

1. *The giver gets more back.* You've heard that the one giving gets more back. You may have heard this statement in regards to the mental and emotional benefits of giving. However, did you also know there are physical benefits?

Evidence of physical benefits is documented in a recent study published in "Psychology and Aging".[22] In this study, 200 hours of volunteering per year correlated to lower blood pressure and greater increases in psychological well-being.[22]

For those of us suffering through a chronic disease, a loss of a loved one, or another crisis, sometimes the best medicine is focusing our mind on something that brings life to someone else. By giving life, it comes back to you, too.

This book only deeply explored two chronic illnesses. You may be experiencing depression, bloating, food sensitivities, eczema, brain fog, or other inflammation conditions. This book will guide you through improving all of those conditions by removing inflammation from your mind, soul, and body, while also giving you tangible step-by-step tools to navigate from getting a proper diagnosis to implementing positive lifestyle changes. So, let's get started.

The process of getting a diagnosis.

The entry of chronic conditions into my life was not on my radar, but it was on God's. He knew that this event would happen. I am so grateful to know that God is in control of all things. He did not create illness (illness was created by sin, environment, stress of this world, genetically modified foods, etc), but we know that God works *all* things together for the good of those who love Him. [23]

I had to rely (and still do every day) on the knowledge that God knows every detail of my body, and He alone is my healer, strength, and source of all wisdom.

Since I was diagnosed with POTS in July 2016 (via a Tilt Test), I have probably seen about 20 doctors. Through prayer, I asked God for discernment and wisdom about the advice the doctors provided.

The process of getting a diagnosis of a chronic condition can be discouraging because the symptoms can vary vastly between individuals.

This journey will have ups and downs - differing opinions and the lack of a solution can lead to fear, uncertainty, and doubt in your mind. These doctors are not God and will likely not conclusively know what is wrong with you. Doctors are simply using experience coupled with certain tests to eliminate possible causes. Then, one-by-one, causes are removed and the most common set of potential causes (based on your symptoms) are identified until they find the root cause. Doctors are not all-knowing (only God is), so when you get discouraged keep your eyes on the only true Healer, and continue to work through the process with your team of doctors.

With your mind prepared for the process ahead:

(1) See more than one doctor.

Do not rely on the opinion of one doctor. This is your life, and you only get one time around this merry-go-round. Your life is worth the cost to ensure you know what you are treating before you start on a path of treatment (one which you may be on for weeks or years). Make sure you are treating the right condition.

Not all doctors are equally qualified, have the time in their schedule to find answers for your unique condition, or desire to be on a journey of healing with you (reviewing how your daily quality of life is affected with each supplement, vitamin, or prescription change).

If two doctors disagree, seek the opinion of a third doctor. Once you've been diagnosed you may be on medication for years, which could have serious side effects. It's worth the investment of time to visit multiple doctors.

(2) Interview your Doctor.

Doctors may be aware of a condition, but that does not mean they have treated patients with that condition. Ask how many patients they have treated for your exact condition. Be specific, ask, "How many patients with this type of condition do you see per week?"

The doctors that are seeing less, are quicker to get into, but are less qualified. You may need to see someone with less experience while being on the waiting list for a doctor who sees 5+ patients a week with your same condition. That's okay. See the less experienced doctor while you are on the waiting list to see the more experienced doctor. You want multiple opinions anyhow.

When I was first diagnosed with POTS, I was able to see a doctor with less experience, who at least knew to get me on salt tablets. This made a huge difference. I went from not being able to care for my toddler to being able to enjoy taking him to the park and playing with him.

But after two months on a waiting list to see an in-demand neurologist, Dr. Geoffrey Sheean with Scripps Coastal Medical Center in La Jolla, California, with strong POTS experience (sees 5+ patients per week), the level of care has dramatically improved.

Dr. Sheean provided insights on other tests to conduct to ensure my body was getting the nutrients it needed to function optimally. He identified vitamins my body was not absorbing, put me on the leaky gut diet, and confirmed the diagnosis of POTS with additional specialized tests.

My health continued to improve after a six-month waiting list for Dr. Thomas Ahern, a cardiologist at Scripps Coastal Medical Center in La Jolla, CA and national expert in POTS.

It truly takes a team.

(3) Keep a binder of test results ("Medical Journal").

We'd like to believe doctors read all your test results before your consultation; this is usually not the case. Therefore, print your own copies of all blood work and doctor visit notes. The nurse will give these to you after each visit if you request them. Bring these with you and read them with your doctor during your visit.

Also, provide each care provider with the lab results and opinions of other medical professionals you've seen thus far.

Lastly, keep a daily journal of your symptoms and their degree of severity. This will allow your doctor to quickly digest the progression or deterioration of symptoms in relation to changes you are making in your medications and diet.

Here is an example of my symptom journal in July 2016:

For a blank Symptom Journal, please go to www.amongme.com/resources.

(4) Have a health advocate.

It is hard to have clarity when you don't feel good, especially if you have an autoimmune or other condition with a symptom of brain fog. It is an emotional time, and it may be difficult to remember everything discussed during your doctor visit. If possible, bring someone with you to each appointment. It is useful to have the same person walk through this process with you - someone to advocate on your behalf when you are too tired, emotional, forgetful, or sick. Sometimes you'll want to give up —your advocate can remind you of how you felt when you started and things are getting better (even if slowly).

Where do I start?

While God is the only true healer, He has gifted certain individuals with the intelligence of medicine. It is important to have a team of health care advocates to support you. Use the above process to screen out health care professionals that won't be able to be in a long journey with you. When you've found the ones that are willing to dedicate the time and energy required, build your team.

There are a variety of specialists that may be needed on your team depending on your unique symptoms and diagnosis (in most cases you'll need more than one specialist). The health care professions you may need on your team may include:
1. General Practitioner (a medical practitioner whose practice is not limited to any specific branch of medicine or class of diseases)
2. Cardiologist (heart)
3. Gastroenterologist (digestive)

4. Endocrinologist (hormone and metabolic systems)
5. Hematologist (blood)
6. Immunologist (immune system)
7. Rheumatologist (musculoskeletal disease and systemic autoimmune conditions)
8. Pulmonologists (respiratory system)
9. Nephrologist (kidneys)
10. Orthopedics (musculoskeletal system [bones, joints, nerves, etc.])

Medical physicians (above) diagnose and treat conditions and illnesses by examining patients, taking medical histories, prescribing medications, and ordering, performing, and interpreting diagnostic tests. Usually the expertise required to treat one organ or system (ie: heart) is not knowledge that you would get from another doctor. Therefore, you'll likely need to see a different domain doctor for each organ or system you think may be showing symptoms. However, it is imperative that you do two things:

1. Keep your Medical Journal up-to-date with each doctor's notes, blood work, medications, and symptoms. Bring it with you to each visit, and make sure each doctor reviews it with you. Your symptoms may change over time. Don't assume the treatment of care you start with will remain the same.

2. Have one MVP on your team, one doctor that helps you keep track of your symptoms over time, and is consistent throughout this journey with you. The MVP may come from your current list of doctors; however, usually it is a General Practitioner or a Natural or Integrated Medicine Doctor.

What is a natural or integrated medicine doctor?

A Natural doctor operates under the belief that the body will heal itself. Natural medicine emphasizes prevention and the self-healing process through the use of natural therapies.

An Integrated Medicine doctor is healing-oriented treatment that takes account of the whole person (body, mind, and spirit), including all aspects of diet and lifestyle. It emphasizes the therapeutic relationship and makes use of all appropriate therapies, both conventional and alternative.

With diet, exercise, prayer, and worship being a large part of the healing process, having a coach that understand the potential of these components toward your ultimate health is critical.

Many times, autoimmune symptoms can be caused by a lack of essential vitamins and nutrients your body needs to function properly (or an excess of foods that ignite inflammation in your system). This is exactly why we need an advocate measuring vitamin levels and food sensitivities - a special focus of natural and integrated medicine health care professionals.

Don't be discouraged by how many doctors you have to visit. Know this upfront, it is a process. You are interviewing them to be on your team and no one will care more about your health than you. Find the right team of champions to weather the storms ahead together. This may mean you'll have to stop seeing a doctor who is not listening to you or spending adequate time to hear your changing symptoms. That is okay. Research additional specialists and schedule your next appointment.

If you live in an area with limited healthcare providers, do consider a bi-annual or quarterly visit to a larger urban area with more options of doctors. Although inconvenient and potentially costly, having an expert you can call, e-mail, and consult with is vital.

Now that we've uncovered the root causes of chronic conditions, lifestyle changes for immediate treatment, and how to build your medical support team with the right players, let's dive into the 4 Gs of Healing and commence your journey of deeper healing.

PART ONE

4 Gs of Healing

GLOW
DIET AND EXCERCISE

Romans 12:1 (NIV)
"Therefore, I urge you, brothers and sisters, in view of God's mercy, to offer your bodies as a living sacrifice, holy and pleasing to God-this is your true and proper worship."

'''''''''''''''''''''''''''

Exercise

Having an autoimmune or chronic disease can make exercise seem unrealistic at times. Your body may be fatigued, joints aching, organs not performing optimally, and sometimes mental health might be suffering too. Normally, that is not the description of someone about to hit the gym for a cardio and weight workout.

Even if your heart desires to be able to physical perform 'like you used to,' your body may be protesting even getting out of bed. It is hard, but it is not impossible.

When POTS first hit me with fatigue and faintness so intense that I could not get out of bed for 2 weeks, I thought I would never run again. There should be a new word in the dictionary for fatigue related to a chronic illness that means, 'complete body shutdown'.

I eventually got up to shower, and then got back to the gym about a month later. My "workouts" started slow with ten minutes on the bike on level three. Then slowly, as my body started to heal, I got back to my previous ability to run six miles and lift weights. It was a slow process. I just showed up every day (and usually I felt better after I did, but honestly, some days I did not). I trusted the research that shows being active is important for those with a chronic health condition,[37] and kept going, knowing that God would give me the strength to do what I needed to do for that day. I know that the consistent workouts were instrumental in my body healing and regaining my life as symptoms were pressed into a state of remission.

Now, most days are good days. However, I still need to properly nourish my body to ensure I start each day with proper hydration and nourishment. Each morning, I have protein, carbs (that agree with my body), and a drink I call "natural electrolyte delight" which a friend, fitness legend, and protein nutritional supplement guru, Jay Robb, introduced to me (www.jayrobb.com). It includes juice from two limes, big pinch of salt, and eight ounces of water – using sparkling water makes it more fun.

I also need to be intentional to get my body in motion: cleaning out the toxins in my body and jump-starting my lymphatic system. For me, salt is instrumental prior to a workout because of POTS.

For many people with chronic health conditions, moderate, low-impact exercise can vastly improve their quality of daily life. I know this because I've lived its truth in my own life.

Also, because studies show those that exercise and have a chronic condition enjoy a better quality of life than those who do not exercise.[37]

Physical activity is especially important in managing chronic conditions for several reasons. Not only is exercise necessary for proper detoxification of the lymphatic system and to reduce inflammation throughout the body, it also has many other benefits. Exercise:

1. increases brain sensitivity for the hormones serotonin and norepinephrine.
2. boosts endorphin production (a natural painkiller).
3. supports fast metabolism.
4. helps maintain muscle mass and weight loss.
5. builds and maintains strong muscles and bones.
6. increases energy levels, even for those with chronic fatigue and other serious diseases like cancer and multiple sclerosis.
7. reduces risk of chronic disease.
8. provides antioxidant protection and promotion of blood flow, which can protect your skin and delay signs of aging.
9. can stimulate the production of hormones that can enhance the growth of brain cells, improving brain health and memory.
10. improves sleep quality providing a feeling of energy throughout the day.
11. can help those with chronic pain reduce their pain and improve the quality of their lives, including chronic lower back pain, fibromyalgia, and chronic soft tissue shoulder disorder and a variety of other conditions.
12. has been proven to boost sex drive.[38]

Exercise routines for those with an autoimmune condition have a different objective than those training for a big race or other athletic competition. Those with autoimmune are conditioning for a better quality of life for a lifetime. There is no end to this quest. Therefore, have fun with it. Change your routines and find ways to exercise that you enjoy.

Doing a mixture of aerobic and muscle-strengthening activities three to five times a week for 30 to 60 minutes is a good target for enjoying the above-mentioned benefits and increase mental health. Exercising just once a week will not increase endurance and doesn't help maintain muscle flexibility.

However, you may need to start with daily gentle stretching and a short daily walk if tolerated without exhaustion. Remember to start slow. You have time to ramp up. It's more important to build endurance slowly. At first it may seem small, but a small walk is a foundational stone to where you are going.

Here are some tips to get started:

1. *Listen to your body; know what works for you.* Chronic conditions have a variety of symptoms, and you know yours best. Start slowly with the introduction of workouts and progress to more challenging ones, as your body is ready. Some days will be harder than others, and if you miss a day because of a flare, that's okay, just get back to the gym or workout routine the next day.

2. *Connect with your team.* Discuss your workout plans with your medical professional team. If you are not sure where to start, make an appointment with a personal trainer to help build a custom

workout plan that fits your ability, condition, and incorporates types of exercise you enjoy.

3. *Select low-impact exercises.* Low-impact activities are easier on your joints. Consider exercises like swimming, pilates, yoga, walking on the treadmill (incline while holding on is a great workout), weight training, low-impact circuit training, and step climbing.

The 6-Week 4 Gs Healing Plan empowers you with a step-by-step program to get started. Of course, before starting any diet, exercise, or lifestyle plan, you should consult with your medical physician.

Diet

The US Centers for Disease Control and Prevention (CDC) estimates that half of Americans suffer from at least one chronic illness, while such diseases cause 70% of US deaths every year.[24]

Even chronic diseases among children have quadrupled since the 1960s. Something is inherently wrong with the food that we are consuming.[25]

Our society has gone from eating foods that were carefully grown and harvested with thoughtful cooking to eating processed convenient foods that are mass produced with little nutritional value and packed with artificial ingredients.

Conventional medicine is now seeing numerous patients coming in with chronic illness, and doctors don't have a cure for these varied conditions besides prescriptions to manage the symptoms. Rarely is conventional medicine providing care treatments for the root cause.

An alternative approach is needed in cooperation with conventional medicine to diagnose and treat the root cause.

Conventional medicine is very useful in identifying the diagnosis. Partnering conventional medicine diagnosis and care with the root healing approach of functional and integrated medicine is very powerful. This partnership empowers you with comprehensive monitoring of your blood work, supplements, vitamins, diet, and medications as the formula will change as you begin to heal.

It is rarely one element alone that triggered a chronic condition, and therefore, the solution is usually more complex than one simple step. Eating and workout habits are critical, but so are the state of your relationships, career, stress level, soul health, and mental peace.

In this section we focus on diet, but please note that intentional focus on all four aspects of the 4 Gs of Healing is critical. We are complex beings and all four areas work in conjunction and affect the other. You will only be as healthy as your least healthy 4G of Healing (Gratitude, Glow, Giving and Grace).

Vitamins and minerals.

Talk to your functional or integrated medical doctor about taking additional omega-3 fatty oils as such has been found to help chronic inflammation.[26] Also, leaky gut can cause malabsorption of needed vitamins and minerals.[27] Ask your doctor for a full blood work panel to see what vitamins and minerals you may be deficient in, including but not limited to vitamin B1, vitamin B6, vitamin B12, vitamin D, folate, iron, vitamin K, magnesium, selenium, zinc, and a full metabolic panel. Having a deficit of just one vitamin or mineral can cause serious symptoms. If you are vitamin deficient, you may feel fatigued, experience neuropathies or muscle pain, and other related symptoms. For example, just vitamin K plays an important role in bone and brain function, healthy metabolism, and protecting against cancer. Deficiency in vitamin K can lead to heart disease, weakened bones, tooth decay, and cancer.[28]

Also, have your heavy metal toxicity tested and check your amino acids. Often those with leaky gut syndrome may be deficient in one or more of these essential elements.

Lastly, if you have any thyroid concerns, have your TSH, TPO antibodies, TG antibodies, T3 Free, and T4 Free labs drawn.

Remove inflammation from gut.

70 to 80% of the immune system is in your intestinal tract.[2] So common sense would tell us that in order to heal our immune system, we must heal our gut. This includes removing all gluten - a protein found in wheat, rye, barley, and many other grains contributes to gut inflammation and may cause leaky gut or an autoimmune condition.

Leaky gut (intestinal permeability) is a condition that happens as a result of intestinal tight-junction malfunction. "Tight junctions" are the gateways between your intestines and what is passed into your blood stream. Tight junctions keep undesirable inflammatory agents out of your blood stream such as toxins, undigested foods, and microbes.[29]

A common symptom of leaky gut is food sensitivity. Due to the intestinal permeability and toxins entering the blood steam, the immune system produces various antibodies that attack antigens in certain foods, especially gluten, and dairy. However, those antibodies may also attack proteins in foods that look similar to those in gluten and dairy such as corn, oats, and rice.[31] Therefore, it is important to follow a proper elimination diet to determine which foods are causing inflammation in your body.

Elimination Diet:

There are a few names for the elimination diet that include autoimmune Paleo diet and autoimmune protocol ("AIP") diet; although, the substance and process of these programs are all very similar. Before you start any diet, you should consult with a medical professional.

PHASE 1: 6-8 weeks

Foods that are not allowed:
- Nuts (ex: all nuts and oils from nuts)
- Seeds and herbs from seeds (ex: chia, sesame, flax, cumin, sesame oil, etc.).
- Beans and legumes (ex: green beans, soy in all forms, peas, black, etc.)
- Grains (ex: corn, wheat, buckwheat, rice, millet, amaranth, rye, spelt, teff, kamut, quinoa)
- Dried fruit

- Dairy (ex: yogurt, milk, cheese, etc.)
- All processed foods
- Alcohol
- Chocolate
- Eggs
- Guar gum, lecithin, xanthan gum
- Nightshade vegetables (ex: tomatoes, potatoes, peppers, eggplant, paprika, mustard seeds)
- No vegetable oils (ex: palm oil)
- Culinary herbs from seeds (ex: mustard, cumin, coriander, fennel, cardamom, nutmeg, dill seed, caraway, etc.)
- Tapioca[36]

Foods that are allowed:
- Vegetables (besides nightshades)
- Fruits (limit to 15-20 grams of fructose per day)
- Fats (ex: Coconut oil, olive oil, avocados, lard, bacon fat, cultured ghee [casein and lactose free])
- Coconut products (ex: manna, creamed coconut, coconut milk – with no added guar gum, shredded coconut)
- Bone broth
- Grass-fed meats, poultry, and seafood
- Non-seed herbal teas
- Green tea
- Vinegars (ex: apple cider, coconut, red wine, and balsamic)
- Binders (ex: grass-fed gelatin and arrowroot starch)[36]

Here is a web URL with a complete list of all foods from Paleomom.com: https://www.thepaleomom.com/start-here/the-autoimmune-protocol/ [32]

If you've been on the elimination diet for 6-8 weeks and have not seen any improvement, you should consult your medical professional as you may need to be tested for other areas of healing such as SIBO (small intestine bacteria overgrowth), heavy metal toxicity, viral inflammation or you may simply need more time on the elimination diet.

PHASE 2: Reintroduction of foods.

If you have an autoimmune condition or leaky gut, Amy Meyers, M.D. recommends that you never reintroduce gluten and cow dairy back to your diet.[33]

She also recommends not reintroducing artificial colors, artificial preservatives, artificial sweeteners, dyes, genetically modified foods, high fructose corn syrup, hydrogenated fat, and trans fats. And, avoid high amounts of alcohol, caffeine, grains, legumes, and sugar.[33]

It is also recommended that one does not go back to high amounts of salt, but James DiNicolantonio in the *Salt Fix* outlines why salt is in fact beneficial (unless you have a condition that makes it difficult for you to processing salt).[34] It is certainly the case for those with POTS that increasing salt consumption is actually benefical.[35]

If you attempt to reintroduce a food unsuccessfully, you may try again in a month or two as your gut continues to heal.

Also, test your antibodies and inflammation with your medical professional as healing symptoms may not be obvious. Test and compare markers before you start the elimination diet and after adding back eliminated food.

However, if you are on immune suppressant medications, you may not notice lab marker changes.

As you heal, you may be able to work with your doctors to see if reducing or eliminating immunosuppressive drugs is possible.

Foods to test reintroducing include: eggs (start with egg yolks and then test egg whites separately), eggplant, goat dairy, peppers, potatoes, sheep dairy, seed-based spices, and tomatoes. Regarding eggs, if you are not able to tolerate them, ensure you are purchasing pastured, soy-free, wheat-free eggs.

Other foods to reintroduce that are less likely to be challenging are seeds, nuts, alcohol (small quantities), coffee (small quantities occasionally), and cocoa or chocolate.

Reintroduce one of the above listed foods at a time. Eat the selected food three times a day for two days. If you sense a reaction, stop eating that food immediately. Possible symptoms of inflammation or sensitivity are listed in Week 7 of the 6-Week 4 Gs of Healing Plan.

Once you've tested a food for two days, return to the elimination diet for three days to neutralize your system before testing the next food item.

Then, once you've tested each food separately for two days and returned three days back to the elimination diet, you can add back in all the foods that did not cause an inflammation or sensitivity response.

There are a number of great resources to educate you on why the elimination diet works; however, I recommend you see a functional or integrated medical professional to help measure your inflammation and specific diet plan and supplements for your specific condition.

GRATITUDE
INTENTIONAL THOUGHTS TRANSFORM

Philippians 4:6 (NIV)
"Do not be anxious about anything but in every situation,
by prayer and petition, with thanksgiving, present
your requests to God."

˙ ˙

What's happening in your life?

Chances are that when your doctor asks the question, "What brings you here today?" and your answer includes an inflammation situation, there is an underlying deeper issue.[39] What is happening in your life? Your marriage? Your school or job? Your finances? Your children's lives? Your plans for the future?

Peeling this onion will reveal inflammatory situations worth examining. Are you in the midst of a divorce? Does your career align with your deepest spiritual principles? Are you worried about losing your job? Are you withholding forgiveness toward anyone?

For complete physical healing, these emotional inflammatory situations need to be addressed in addition to their physical manifestations. Many people ruin their health and their lives by taking the poison of bitterness, resentment, and mercilessness.

Dr. Caroline Leaf, a cognitive neuroscientist with a PhD in Communication Pathology and a BSc in Leogopedics and Audiology, shares that "75% to 95% of the illnesses that plague us today are a direct result of our thought life. What we think about affects us physically and emotionally."[40]

If you don't believe that dealing with these issues will help your physical condition, why not try it? Try working on just one of those situations and see if it doesn't improve your physical health as well. If inflammation can be removed from your body without having to take medication, isn't it worth trying?

"In anger, his master handed him over to the jailers to be tortured, until he should pay back all he owed. This is how my heavenly Father will treat each of you unless you forgive your brother and sister from your heart." (Matthew 18:24-25 NIV)

The goal of the 4Gs of Gratitude is to reduce inflammation from all aspects of your life. So, let's get started on healing your thought-life.

Replace toxic thoughts with life-giving scripture and truth.

Remember, everything you do is first a physical thought in your brain. You think, and then you act. Hence if your thinking is positive, then your actions and communications are positive. The same is true if your thinking is toxic. Be intentional about what thoughts you allow to take up residence in your mind.

For example, if you think you will never get well or that your marriage is done, that thought will lead you to behave in a way that reflects that dominate belief. However, if you choose to speak hope and positive truth over that thought, you will start to reprogram the way you think and behave toward that same situation. Instead of giving mental space to thoughts that your marriage is over, you can thoughtfully decide to replace that undesired thought with a belief that your relationship may be in a rough season, but it is not over. You can purposefully focus on the reasons you fell in love and who your spouse can and will be in the future. When entering a room, instead of you ignoring your partner, your first reaction could be to smile and offer a comment of gratefulness for something about them.

Change happens in a moment when you decide to change your thoughts. The results from that decision may, at first, be small and some may dramatically impact a circumstance, belief, or relationship immediately. Either way, when you are intentional about meditating on those thoughts that are positive, true, and scripture-based, you will see effects in your mental, physical, and spiritual health.

Here are some scriptures and life-giving thoughts to intentionally meditate upon.

- I can do all this through him who gives me strength. (Philippians 4:13 NIV)
- I will not die but live, and will proclaim what the Lord has done. (Psalm 118:17)
- The Lord will fight for you; you need only to be still. (Exodus 14:14 NIV)
- Finally, brothers and sisters, whatever is true, whatever is noble, whatever is right, whatever is pure, whatever is lovely, whatever is

admirable – if anything is excellent or praiseworthy – think about such things. (Philippians 4:8 NIV)

- For the Spirit God gave us does not make us timid, but gives us power, love and self-discipline. (2 Timothy 1:7 NIV)
- And the peace of God, which transcends all understanding, will guard your hearts and minds in Christ Jesus. (Philippians 4:7 NIV)
- Do not be anxious about anything but in every situation, by prayer and petition, with thanksgiving, present your requests to God. (Philippians 4:6 NIV)
- Cast all your anxiety on him because he cares for you. (1 Peter 5:7)
- God is our refuge and strength, an ever-present help in trouble. (Psalm 46:1)
- Brothers and sisters, I do not consider myself yet to have taken hold of it. But one thing I do: Forgetting what is behind and straining toward what is ahead, I press on toward the goal to win the prize for which God has called me heavenward in Christ Jesus. (Philippines 3:13-14)
- Just because you decide to replace a toxic thought does not mean that it will be replaced the first or the one-hundredth time. But if you are consistent for 21 days, you can rebuild that thought and the emotions tied to it with a new thought-pattern.

Replace toxic actions with life-giving approaches.

As you replace toxic thoughts with scripture and life-giving thoughts, your actions will automatically start to follow. For example, if you think about ice cream long enough, within that same day you will likely stop at the supermarket to buy ice cream. Your actions follow your thoughts.

In addition, here are some intentional actions that can reduce situational inflammation from our lives.

Offer Forgiveness Quickly and Avoid Bitterness

According to Karen Swartz, M.D., director of the Mood and Disorders Adult Consultation Clinic at John Hopkins, "There is an enormous physical burden to being hurt and disappointed."[42]

John Hopkins further states in their article "Forgiveness: Your Health Depends on It" that, "Chronic anger puts you in a flight-or-fight mode, which results in numerous changes in heart rate, blood pressure, and immune response. Those changes, then, increase the risk of depression, heart disease, and diabetes, amongst other conditions. Forgiveness, however, calms stress levels, leading to improved health."[43]

Forgiveness is not just stating forgiveness or deciding not to think negative thoughts. "It is an active process in which you make a conscious decision to let go of negative feelings whether the person deserves it or not," Swartz says.[42]

Steps to Deep Forgiveness:

1. *Reflect.* Remember the event including your emotions and perceptions.

2. *Empathize.* Consider the other person's emotions and perceptions. Consider why they acted the way they did or if they were expressing

an unmet need or expectation. Perhaps their childhood contributed to their action.

3. *Prayer.* Ask God to forgive you for holding hardheartedness toward this person in your heart. Pray that He would fill your heart with compassion and forgiveness for this person. Pray that God would bless and grow this person to know Him better. Release that person to God in Jesus's name.

4. *Forgive Deeply.* No one is perfect. We all make mistakes – small and big. The Lord forgave us of all our sins and commands that we forgive others of theirs. Remember who you were before you met Christ and all He has done for you. The sins of any person against us can never compare to our sins against our Father. If the person doesn't deserve forgiveness, forgive because it hampers your relationship with your Heavenly Father, and forgiveness knocks down that barrier and gives you emotional freedom.

5. *Let go of expectations.* An apology may not change or reconcile a relationship. That person may not apologize back. You or that person may not want an on-going relationship or perhaps healthy boundaries need to be set going forward that change the dynamics of the relationship. That is okay if the change is done in an effort to connect in healthy ways and not to punish the other person. Forgiveness does not always mean reconciliation or going back to the way things were before. "As far as it is up to you, live at peace" Romans 12:18 (NIV).

6. *Forgive yourself.* The act of forgiving includes yourself. For example, if you had an affair, you will self-sabotage your marriage or another area of your life if you don't forgive yourself. Confess your feelings (guilt, anger, disappointment, etc.) to a close friend, counselor, or pastor so they can pray with you. Ask God for forgiveness and know that His grace is sufficient to cover all of our sins.

Address Ongoing Relationship or Work Tensions

Make a plan to address those parts of your life that cause you the most friction (aka relationship or situational inflammation).

Make a list of the top two to five personal or professional relationships or situations that cause friction in your life. In families as well as in commercial settings, frictions arise from the interdependent relationships required in forward coordination amongst diverse experiences, opinions and beliefs. So, the question is how can we change the dynamic of the coordination? Here are a few approaches:

1. *Change the dance.* If there is a pattern, whereas your partner does or says something to trigger a negative response from you, change your response. If you would have normally responded with a quick-tongue comment, instead laugh and give them a huge bear hug. Your change in response may seem unnatural but it will change the rhythm and atmosphere in your home.

2. *Be truthful in kindness.* If your colleague is continuously late on deadlines causing you to work late, you could ask them to lunch.

Select an atmosphere that is calm and if possible, where you can share a meal. Express gratitude for a positive attribute of your working relationship and how you want to ensure that your working relationship always remains open and as enjoyable as it is today. Explain that out of respect for your relationship and your colleague, that you want to bring to their attention how they were late on Tuesday's and Thursday's deadlines, which caused you to work late and miss your daughter's recital. Acknowledge that you know your colleague would not purposely intend to put you in that situation and that is why you want to brainstorm together how deadlines could be set so that you both can work normal hours.

3. *Ask for a favor, show gratitude.* "He that has once done you a kindness will be more ready to do you another, than he whom you yourself have obliged" – Benjamin Franklin.[44]

When habitual friction is experienced with a colleague, you could ask them for a favor. If someone from another department at work judges your work unfairly, you can ask them to show you how to use a new software application. Then, express authentic and humble gratitude to them for assisting you. People grow to like people for whom they do kind things.

We are Human, Seek God for Help

Let's face it: some of these mental and behavioral changes will be hard. Your heart may be so cold or hardened toward someone that it causes anxiety to even think about forgiving them. What we cannot do in the natural, God can do in the supernatural. Start praying for them and ask God to change your heart for them. God will meet you. He loves us and wants us to experience emotional freedom and healing.

Therefore, each time the negative thought pattern comes up, hand it over to God. Let God handle the situation, and pray for the person. Pray that God will give you a forgiving heart and ponder on good attributes or times you had with that person. If all you can think of is that they have a nice smile - focus on that. Then, let them go to God. Holding on to the negative thought pattern will only hurt you. The other person doesn't feel a thing, but your physical, mental, and soul health are being hurt now. Let it go. If you don't, that person will continue to steal your life from you, as your health will follow your negative thought patterns.

Choose forgiveness. Choose freedom. Choose whole health and energy.

Cultivate an Attitude of Gratitude

Get up every morning. Before you get out of bed and meditate on this truth:

"This is the day the Lord has made. We will rejoice and be glad in it." (Psalm 118:24 NKJV)

Be honest, the majority of us don't get out of bed flooded with immediate thoughts of gratitude and joy. Instead, our first thought might be, "I just want one day to sleep in" or "I have to go to work today and that presentation is due" or "Why do I have to get up with the baby? I am always the one who gets up."

Cultivating an attitude of gratitude requires an intentional practice consistently executed every day.

I like to start each day with quiet time with the Lord. I prefer an hour, but with a toddler and husband to get off to school and work respectively, sometimes such time is only 15 minutes.

If I jump right into prayer, I find that my prayers are often one-sided (me talking) and full of prayer requests. God help me to...

On those days, I meet briefly with God but I usually don't experience God.

The far better are the days when I intentionally cultivate an attitude of gratitude and praise before the Lord. Then I find myself resting in His wisdom and guidance and my day is more peaceful (even if there are storms).

Over the years, I have found the following simple three-step practice has helped me cultivate an attitude of gratitude and praise.

1. *Start with prayer.* Thank God for this day and that I have air in my lungs. Thank Him for those in my life that I get the opportunity to serve and love today. Thank God for the daily provision and abundance He has blessed our family with. Ask forgiveness from those I offended and from God. Forgive those who have hurt me intentionally or unintentionally. And pray for protection for our family and relatives in the name of Jesus Christ.

2. *Daily Gratitude Journal.* I have found that writing out five things I am grateful for today, focuses my heart and day on what is important. I

am a more patient mother when my son doesn't want to get in his car seat when I just thanked God for the honor of being his mother.

3. *Daily Word.* Personally, I like to write out the Word in my journal. I use the Student Bible, as there is a great resource in the back of the Bible, including scriptures identified by topic. So, if I am in a season where I need encouragement, I look for scriptures related to encouragement. You can also find excellent devotionals around seasons of life. I would caution against using Google to find scriptures, as the Internet has too many distractions that could take your mind away from God and the Word.

At www.amongme.com/resources you an access a free download of the Gratitude Journal. This resource is intended to provide you another instrument for experiencing God; however, the ultimate intent is to experience God. So, if you find another method works better for you, please do it.

GIVE

Proverbs 11:25 (NIV)
"A generous person will prosper; whoever refreshes others will be refreshed."

, ,

What is the purpose of your life?

Without a meaning to set your mind about accomplishing, your mind will default to the loudest immediate circumstance or physical symptom. You will begin to focus on every physical symptom and experience a loss of control in your life as you attempt to cure every symptom. This endless mental downward spiral will manifest into living in fear most of the time. Personally, I have experienced this type of daily fear, and it robs you of enjoying life each day.

Instead, intentionally focus on what you can do versus what you can't do or what you fear. And what you can do exceeds your physical ability. Raise your level of thinking to not only what you can do but also what God can do through you. "I can do all this through him who gives me strength" (Philippians 4:13).

Thinking about what you can do and whom you can add value to (bless) will improve your sense of wellness, your actual physical health, and your relationships.

Cultivate an attitude of gratitude.

First, focus on what you can do.

Start each day by cultivating an attitude of gratitude for all the things you can do, the people in your life, and the hope found in the Scriptures. Life is not perfect and your physical capabilities may have changed dramatically, but there are still some things you can do. If you can't get out of bed, you can still be grateful that you can bring hope to others who may be experiencing a similar ailment via online blogs and forums.

Your life is not about you. You were created to be part of a community and to bring joy to others around you. God designed you uniquely with certain gifts and talents. The ecosystem of your existence will be a better place when you spend less time pondering the symptoms of your condition and replace that mental real estate with how to offer grace, encouragement, or a helping hand in the lives of others.

What is your purpose?

You were distinctively designed by God to live a life that glorifies Him by loving and serving others. It is when you are aligned with the original intent for which life was breathed into you that you feel the greatest level of satisfaction and inner peace because you are doing that for which the Designer created you.

We marvel at the beauty of nature and often feel close to God when we are surrounded by nature (His creation). A cloud is beautiful for it was created for specific purpose. It operates and performs that purpose perfectly. It is in that perfect execution that God's glory is witnessed, and we feel closer to Him by seeing it. Humans will never operate perfectly as God gave us freedom of will. However, it is when we operate as closely as we can to that original design that beauty is seen. Others see it and it stands out: they are drawn to the beauty. Our souls feel it, and we experience a peace and joy that surpasses our own understanding.

What would those closest to you say is your driving force of life? What do you want it to be?

If your driving force is to cure your symptoms, you'll live a fearful and discontent life. If your driving force is to bring healing and hope to others who are experiencing chronic conditions, you will gain a sense of accomplishment and joy each time someone is helped along their journey. Be clear, I am not saying not to focus on healing. The 4 Gs of Healing are designed for you to spend mental and physical time each day focused on healing -- just don't allow curing your condition to become the dominant purpose of your life.

You need a purpose for getting well. If you had perfect health today, what would you use it for?

Would you focus on your relationships (spouse, children, parents, colleagues, or distant relatives)? Would you contribute to society (feeding the homeless, rescuing abused animals, protecting vulnerable youth, or serving orphans)? Would you focus on simply bringing kind words and a smile to each person you encounter in a day?

UnitedHealth Group commissioned a national survey of 3,351 adults and found that the overwhelming majority of participants reported feeling mentally and physically healthier after a volunteer experience.[45]

- 76% of people who volunteered in the last 12 months said that volunteering has made them feel healthier.
- 94% of people who volunteered in the last 12 months said that volunteering improved their mood.
- 78% of them said that volunteering lowered their stress levels.
- 96% reported that volunteering enriched their sense of purpose in life.
- 80% of them feel like they have control over their health.
- ~25% of them reported that their volunteer work has helped them manage a chronic illness by keeping them active and taking their minds off of their own problems.
- Volunteers have better personal scores than non-volunteers on nine well-established measures of emotional wellbeing including personal independence, capacity for rich interpersonal relationships, and overall satisfaction with life.
- Volunteering also improved their mood and self-esteem.[45]

What kinds of proactive acts can you do to improve the quality of other's lives?

When more of your thoughts and hours are focused on others and less on your symptoms, your sense of purpose and control grows and fear shrinks. What flourishes in fear's place is a sense of vitality and joy.

GRACE
HE IS OUR STRENGTH

Philippians 4:4 (NIV)
"Rejoice in the Lord always. I say it again: Rejoice!"

A common response to the question, "How are you?", in the American culture, is "Busy."

Smart phones and email access 24/7 has made us more productive as a society but also more stressed and anxious. God intended for us to experience the peace that transforms all understanding. So, how can we reduce stress and anxiety while still living in our fast-paced culture?

The Lord has provided us some simple steps to balance the stress of this world. The disciples faced stress. While writing the letter of Philippians, Paul was in prison awaiting a horrific execution. That's stress! Yet, even in the midst of that circumstance he wrote one of the most joyful books of the Bible. He wrote, "rejoice in the Lord always, I say it again: rejoice!" (Philippians 4:4 NIV).

Where does such optimism and joy come from? The Lord. Spending quiet time with the Lord in prayer and worship. In prison, Paul had a lot of time to spend in the Lord's presence.

As we explore these simple steps to reducing stress, please do not discount the message because of its simplicity. Know that God is love. God wants his children to have the peace that transcends understanding. Therefore, our loving Father, knowing our weaknesses, provided simple steps so that all His children would be able to experience His peace.

First and foremost, schedule a daily quiet time with the Lord. It may be 15 minutes. It may be an hour. The time is not as important as the daily consistency. Spend time in the Bible. It is alive and active. You will experience God through His Word.

Step 1: Cast your anxiety and worry onto the Lord.

This step sounds so simple but in practice is hard to do when the concern is heavy on our hearts. Often when trouble comes (health crisis, relational discord, etc), it's our tendency to turn inward and think continuously about our burden, question why this happened to us, and get lost in the misery of our situation. In Psalms 3-7 David faces trouble. His own son, Absalom, rebelled against his authority and sought to kill him. David is too practical to say forget about your problems and be positive, which I appreciate. Neither David's nor our circumstances are insignificant or minor. They are real and painful. The best way to deal with them is to face them head on in prayer to God and describe the hurt in detail (just like David did in Psalms 3-7). Without pouring out our thoughts in detail to God, they remain vague thoughts whose shadows feed and grow on fear, uncertainty, and doubt in our mind (and cause manifestations in our physical health). However, the powerful truths of God obtained by the practice of prayer and worship always win over fear, uncertainty, and doubt.

Many of us carry the burdens of yesterday (what we should have done differently, how we were treated unfairly), today, and tomorrow (worries about the future or events outside of our control); however, God only gives us enough grace for today.

To reduce stress, let go of the past and the future. God cares for you. Tell Him your fears and give control to the Creator of the universe. He will have more influence than you and I. Live one day at a time. Of course, be prudent in planning when you have influence on the outcome of tomorrow, but don't enter into worrying over things you have no influence to change. Most of the things we worry about will never happen. So, don't lose the joy of today, worrying about something that will never happen.

In fact, research shows that 85% of what we worry about never happens, and when the 15% actually do, subjects found that they could handle the problem better than they expected or that the situation taught them a lesson worth learning.[46] This means that 97% of what you worry over is either never going to happen or is going to happen but with an outcome better than you expect.[46]

"Who of you by worrying can add a single hour to his life?" (Matthew 6:27 NIV).

"Therefore do not worry about tomorrow, for tomorrow will worry about itself. Each day has enough trouble of its own" (Matthew 6:34 NIV).

Step 2: Pray about everything; meditate on truth.

You created mental real estate by casting your anxiety on the Lord, fill that new empty space with prayer and meditation.

Prayer is the transference of a burden from us to God. We are not God, and the multitude of stressors from daily life will overwhelm us. God delights when we believe in Him to fight for us.

Our problems are not too big for God. He is God. He created the stars in their vastness and brilliance. Can He not handle our fears, doubts, insecurities, and troubles?

"Do not be anxious about anything, but in every situation, by prayer and petition, with thanksgiving, present your requests to God. And the peace of God, which transcends all understanding, will guard your hearts and your minds in Christ Jesus" (Philippians 4:6 – 7 NIV).

Meditate on who God is, who you are in Christ Jesus (righteous and dearly loved by God), and the promises of God in the Bible.

Meditation is intentional thinking. Ponder on the truth. Many of the things we worry about are "what if" scenarios. Deliberately take captive "what if" thoughts and replace them with truth. Keep replacing that anxiety or negativity with truth. At first, you might need to do this every five minutes. Eventually, that old thought or worry will be replaced with a new life-giving thought and truth.

"Finally, brothers, whatever is true, whatever is noble, whatever is right, whatever is pure, whatever is lovely, whatever is admirable - if anything is excellent or praiseworthy - think about such things" (Philippians 4:8 NIV).

Step 3: Be content.

How content are you to stand in the checkout line at the grocery store or airport security?

Do you feel you deserve to get the latest iPhone or drive a certain model of car because of how hard you work?

When was the last time you complained? What did you complain about? If we were honest, for those of us living in America, our last complaint was probably a first-world problem.

Our society has lost the art of being content in a culture of selfies and materialism. We sing in worship, "God is enough for me," but do we practice that in our heart?

There is nothing wrong with working hard; in fact, it's admirable. There is nothing wrong with having nice things. And there is nothing wrong with crying out to God with our desires and complaints. He can handle it.

However, discontentment combined with working for the acquisition of material goods brings heaviness into our lives. We may become overworked, replacing time we would have spent with God to do more work. Or we may enter into debt to purchase things we can't afford. Or we may complain without finding peace at the end of our lamenting.

"It is better to have only a little, with peace of mind, than be busy all the time" Ecclesiastes 4:6 GN).

Step 4: Trust God in all things.

It is often said that trust is spelled, T-I-M-E. Trust is born out of a personal relationship. The same is true for our ability to trust God. The more time we spend walking with Him and experiencing His grace and consistent nature, the more we trust Him with other areas of our lives.

God is love. He loves us, and each day, He has plans for our good.

So, why do we stress when we have a Father who created the universe and seeks for ways to bless us every day?

We may believe that God will ask us to do something that is uncomfortable. We may not be walking on the protected road he paved for us, but rather running blindly on a dusty trail of our own finding, filled with stones and potholes. Or we may just believe we can handle the circumstance better by our own reason, even if our way is slightly different from the standard of the Bible. For example, does the Bible really state one must forgive all people; surely, that doesn't include people who intentionally hurt or abandoned you, right? Yes, those people too.

Yes, sometimes trusting God and the Word will be uncomfortable. Sometimes you'll have to forgive people you'd rather just avoid. It is impossible to do things we don't want to do out of sheer willpower for a significant period of time. It is by daily grace that He will give you the exact amount of strength needed to act according to His way on that day.

Trust is built when we realize that God marvelously created each of us with specific traits, talents, and callings. He won't ask someone to go to Africa that He didn't already build a desire in his or her heart to be an international missionary. True, He may ask you to do things that require sacrifice or are uncomfortable, but He will also give you the grace and strength to do them at the right time.

God may not have caused your illness or situation, but He will give you the strength to find joy through the journey. Keep your eyes on Him during the storm and have faith that He will use all things for good, and He has a good plan for you.

He is more interested in growing your soul for eternity and saving the souls of those around you than our comfort. This life is but a whisper. The outcome of listening and obeying Him will have eternal benefit and often will bring joy afterwards in your inner soul. The sweet rejoicing of being a daughter or son in the image of your Father will make discomfort short-lived as you bask in His presence.

Each time you go against what you want to do, and trust God to handle a situation His way, you will build deeper trust with God. You will see how situations are handled in ways you would have never expected but for the good. Trust is built by spending time doing things God's way and being in His presence.

Step 5: Gratitude

Keep a Gratitude Journal. Each morning think on purpose about five things you are grateful for and thank God for the blessing of those things in your life. The Gratitude Journal is available at www.amongme.com/resources.

For those of us who are parents, we know how good it feels when our children are grateful for the good gifts we give them. We work hard each day to provide food, safety, and good things for our children. We appreciate when our children are grateful and enjoy the things we worked hard to provide for them. How much more must our Father long to hear our gratefulness?

I know without the intentional practice of being grateful to God for five specific things each day, I start my conversation to him with needs and complaints. I'm not exactly the best coffee companion for God in those moments. But when I start with gratefulness, it changes my heart. When I leave my time of prayer, there may still be areas I would like God to handle but my soul is more peaceful because I recognize He has given me what I need for today.

PART TWO

Healing Plan

Among Me

6-WEEK
4 Gs OF HEALING PLAN

"I am a firm believer in the mind-body interaction and their potential to create
both disease and health. It is obvious to me that the mind can dramatically
influence inflammation, presumably through the medium of chemical messengers –
neuropeptides produced in the brain that interact directly with immune cells, either
activating or suppressing them."
Andrew Weil, M.D., New York Times bestselling author[47]

Plunging into the interaction between your mind and body is at the core of healing. This 6-Week 4 Gs of Healing Plan is designed to guide you through exercises that will enlighten your awareness of both the healthy and toxic interactions as well as reduce inflammation with diet and movement. Each week will expand on the previous week. Therefore, keep the new behaviors from week 1 as you expand additional behaviors in week 2 and on.

Week 1:

Glow- Diet

Some people are able to jump into a full elimination diet to heal a leaky gut condition; however, I've found a more gradual approach to be helpful for long-term sustainability of the elimination diet. I did not feel as deprived when I reduced a few inflammatory foods and added a few new nutrient-rich foods per week.

1. Remove from diet: soda, artificial sweeteners, sugar, and high-glycemic foods (except sugar from fruit), alcohol, soy, gluten, and dairy.

2. Set an appointment with an integrated medical professional to test your vitamin levels, including but not limited to vitamin B1, vitamin B6, vitamin B12, vitamin D, folate, iron, vitamin K, magnesium, selenium, and zinc. Further, have your full metabolic panel drawn along with tests for heavy metal toxicity. Lastly, if you have thyroid concerns, have labs that include TSH, TPO antibodies, TG antibodies, T3 Free, and T4 Free drawn.

3. Start taking fish oil and vitamin C as recommended on the bottle.

4. Start to reduce your coffee intake to one cup a day. Great coffee alternatives are chai tea (decaf) or chicory root tea. My personal favorite is chicory root tea with coconut milk.

5. Add broccoli and bone broth to diet a few times a week. Preferably beef broth.

There are some tasty and creative recipes to experiment with on the below sites; however, a quick Google search for AIP recipes will result in numerous fun meals to tryout.

http://autoimmunewellness.com/recipes/

https://www.amymyersmd.com/recipes/

Glow- Exercise

Your exercise program should be customized for your fitness level. This plan will outline steps for beginner level movement; still, as with all diet and physical exercise programs, you should consult with your medical provider before commencing. For those of you who are already physically active in cardiovascular and weight activities, you may find the 6-Week Workout Calendar and 6-Week Weight & Circuit Routine, available in the Resource section of Amongme.com, more suitable for your fitness goals.

1. Brisk walk or bike 10 minutes each day.
2. 50-body weight squats 3 x week.

Glow- Rest

Quality sleep is as vital to your health as food and water.[48] Sleep affects every type of tissue and system in your body from the brain, heart, and lungs to metabolism, immune function, mood, and disease resistance.[48]

School-age children and teens on average need about 9.5 hours of sleep at night. Most adults need 7-9 hours of sleep per night.[48]

Respecting the circadian rhythm is instrumental in regulating eating behaviors and changes in appetite stimulating hormones, glucose metabolism, and mood. Circadian misalignment is linked to increased risk of cardiovascular disease, diabetes, obesity, cancer, depression, bipolar, schizophrenia, and attention deficit disorders.[49]

If you are having difficulties falling and staying asleep, here are a few things that can help reset your circadian rhythm:

1. Adjust your bedtime
2. Do not nap
3. Avoid blue light from computer and phone screens. Try amber glasses (you can find these on Amazon)
4. Avoid beverages with caffeine and alcohol in the evening
5. Avoid eating heavy meals at least 2 hours before going to sleep

Gratitude:

How do thoughts affect our physical health?

Dr. Caroline Leaf states, "Research shows that around 87% of illness can be attributed to our thought life, and approximately 13% to diet, genetics, and environment. Studies conclusively link more chronic diseases (also known as lifestyle diseases) to an epidemic of toxic emotions in our culture."[50]

Thoughts cause the brain to release neurotransmitters, chemical messengers that communicate with parts of itself and your nervous system. Neurotransmitters are vital in the function of many body functions including hormone, digestion, and emotions regulation.[51]

In fact, there are more than 100 chemical substances produced in the body that have been identified as neurotransmitters.[52]

According to Dr. Caroline Leaf in her book, *Who Switched Off My Brain?*, at any one moment your brain is performing about 400 billion actions and we are only conscious of about 2,000. Each of those 400 billion actions has both a chemical and electrical component responsible for triggering emotions.[50]

For example, when you exercise, your brain releases a specific chemical or neurotransmitters called endorphins, which is one reason movement is a key ingredient in the 4 Gs of Healing program.

Alternatively, when you feel emotions of sadness, fear, uncertainty, guilt, excessive grief, resentment, and hardheartedness, your brain releases different types of chemicals that are harmful to your physical health (especially over time).

For example, anxiety is a reaction to stress that has both psychological and physical features. According to an article by the Harvard Medical School, "The feeling is thought to arise in the amygdala, a brain region that governs many intense emotional responses. As neurotransmitters carry the impulse to the sympathetic nervous system, heart and breathing rates increase, muscles tense, and blood flow is diverted from the abdominal organs to the brain. In the short term, anxiety prepares us to confront a crisis by putting the body on alert. But its physical effects can be counterproductive, causing lightheadedness, nausea, diarrhea, and frequent urination. When it persists, anxiety can take a toll on our mental and physical health."[61]

How do I reprogram my thoughts?

Silence your body by sitting down and removing all electronic influences. Ask God for wisdom as to what thoughts you are repeating to yourself daily. Repeating thoughts over and over is a form of self-hypnosis. These thoughts are real things and will influence your mental and physical health.

Specifically, focus on what is a toxic thought you repeat daily (ie: thoughts of anger, fear, hardheartedness, guilt, shame, or negative thoughts about who you are or what you're capable of). The one you repeat most often is the first thought we want to reprogram.

Write on paper your answers to the following questions in regards to that toxic thought:

1. Why did you adopt this belief or thought?
2. What is the truth?
3. How has this belief or thought held you back from the life (mental and physical) that you'd like to have?
4. If you don't reprogram the impact this belief or thought has had in your life, what will the future look like? How will you feel?
5. If you do reprogram the impact this belief or thought will have in your life, what will your future look like? How will you feel?
6. At some point did this belief or thought serve to protect you? How could you protect yourself in another way without giving more life to this toxic belief or thought?

Feel the emotions tied to these answers so that you can release the pain. If you "put aside" toxic emotions until a more opportune time to deal with them, eventually that box of emotions will spill over and manifest in physical health issues. If these emotions have been stored in your memory for some time, it might be beneficial to speak with a counselor to help you process these stored up emotions.

Feeling your emotions means expressing them in an environment that is safe, accepting, and non-judgmental. This may mean speaking with a counselor or writing a letter, and always prayer. Don't deny your feelings, acknowledge them, and deal with them in as positive way as possible.

Now that you've identified your heaviest toxic thought, how do we reprogram it?

Step One: Prayer. Talk to God as you would a friend, and ask Him to show you truth over this toxic thought and the freedom He desires for you to have. Praise God that He is the one who heals, and ask Him for His understanding, which surpasses our own. Lastly, ask for the strength to take control of your thoughts by His power within you.

If you are specifically dealing with the negative emotion of hardheartedness, here is an example prayer:

> *Dear Lord, I thank You for the power of forgiveness, and I choose to forgive ___<name>_____ who has hurt me. Help me set _____<name>_____ free and release them to You. Help me pray for those who have hurt me. Help me walk in righteousness, peace, and joy, demonstrating Your life here on earth. I choose to forgive others, just as You forgave me. In Jesus' name, amen.*

If you're a Christian carrying guilt around, it's because you're not taking advantage of what Jesus Christ did on the cross. God has given us a way to get rid of guilt. It's called confession. God promises that when we confess, He forgives us instantly, totally, completely, freely, and continuously. Give God your guilt. He wants to forgive you (no matter what you did). If you are not a Christian and would like to accept Christ as your Lord and Savior, see the

Prayer Resource at the back of this book for a specific prayer to invite Jesus into your life.

Step Two: Set Your Mind. Set your mind to consciously take control of your thought life. Examine each thought (and determine if that thought is beneficial to your health) and consciously consider whether to accept that thought as truth into your brain or reject it. It will take intentional work to not allow thoughts to just wander through your mind. You need to pull toxic thoughts into your conscious and wrestle with them.

Step Three: Choose Your Words. The words you speak have powerful programming effectiveness. When you make negative comments, negative chemicals are released. These words are a form of self-hypnosis as they lead to negative emotions and memories. Changing your words to positive words is not enough. You must actually believe what you say. Instead, replace negative words with attitude-adjusting words. To do this:

- Acknowledge that an issue exists or a perceived issue.
- Ask yourself, "Is this thought true?" If not, reject it.
- If it is true, how can you cope with it in as positive way as possible?

Step Four: Proactively Reprogram Toxic Emotions. You identified the greatest toxic thought and reflected on how that toxic thought has affected your life.

Now, write on paper what a more positive, truthful attitude and thought would be to replace that thought.

Next, write down what impact changing your attitude and thought would have on your future happiness. How would changing this pattern affect your happiness and relationship with others?

Lastly, write on the same paper, one thing you can do today to start acting in alignment with this new belief?

Reward yourself each time you successful reject the old thought pattern and choose the new thought pattern. The reward could be small...like a mental high-five to yourself or something larger like a cup of tea. If possible, try to tie a physical action as an anchor to the new thought pattern (ie: smiling really big or saying "yes" out loud). The physical reaction will be something you can start to do to recall your new thought and experience the emotion of successfully changing your thoughts.

For 3-weeks, focus on your greatest toxic thought identified above. Focus on exchanging the negative thought pattern with your new thought pattern by taking daily action.

Journal your experiences and successes each day. Start each day with identifying one proactive action you can take today to reprogram your thought pattern. Experience and reflect on your successes and how that makes you feel. Action and emotion must be tied to the process to get lasting, meaningful results.

Give:

Make it your objective to think of yourself less during the day by intentionally thinking about others. We never know the full extent of another's burdens. Identify one thing you can do for another this week that captures your heart. What you select must be something you authentically desire to do. Here are some ideas:

- Speaking encouragement to a friend who is going through a rough season.
- Baking cookies for (or with) your kids.
- Volunteering for a day at your children's school.
- Expressing gratitude to your teacher for her efforts to impact your and other's lives.
- Telling your mother or father that you appreciate their sacrifices. Be specific.
- Volunteering in the daycare or greeting team at your church.

Grace:

Print out the Gratitude Journal found at www.amongme.com/resources. Start each morning with prayer, your Bible, and this journal (even if you only have 10 minutes). These simple steps will provide you living hope throughout the day by setting your mind on what He can do and not on what is seen.

- **Praise Scripture:** Write out one scripture from the Bible. Key Verses to get you started can be found at www.amongme.com/resources. Praise God for who He is. Ponder on how He is the creator of the stars, sun, and ocean. There is nothing that is impossible for God. He created our bodies and knows every cell in them.
- **Gratitude:** Write 5 things you are grateful for this morning.
- **Thoughts:** Write anything that is revealed to you through prayer, the Word, or any experience you have through this journey.
- **Prayer Requests & Answered Prayers:** The best method I have found for finding hope is to remember all the Lord has done for me. He knows and cares about the details of my days. Keeping a record of

my prayer requests and answered prayers provides me evidence of His engagement in my life activated by prayer. It reminds me that prayer has power and is a great encouragement in times I don't hear from God or feel I am alone in this health battle.

Week 2:

Glow- Diet

Continue the elimination diet and remove the following additional foods: eggs, nuts, seeds, legumes, and nightshade family foods (i.e. tomatoes, potatoes, eggplant, and peppers). Reduce coffee to ½ cup a day.

Add the following foods to your diet: grass-fed organ meats and grass-fed gelatin or collagen.

See the Resource section of Amongme.com for a complete listing of all foods allowed and not allowed on the elimination (a.k.a. AIP Protocol Diet). This resource is produced by Paleomom.com[53] and is also an excellent overview of the purposes of the diet.

Keep a journal of any increase or decrease in the symptoms you experience. You can find a Symptom Journal at www.amongme.com/resources.

Glow- Exercise:

1. Increase brisk walk or bike to 15 minutes per day.
2. 3 sets of 10 abdominal crunches per day
3. 50 body-weight squats 3 times a week

Gratitude:

Continue your Daily Journal and intentional action to reprogram the first toxic thought or belief.

Add at least three minutes a day visualizing yourself acting consistent with your new thought. Feel how you would feel if you were free from that old pattern of thinking and living in the daily hope resulting from your new thought pattern. Experience that emotion and visualize how you would act differently. How would your relationships be improved? How would your health be improved?

Visualization is a powerful technique to gain access to healing. In some cases, visualization could produce complete healing and in some enhance the effectiveness of other treatments.

In the Psychology Today article, *Seeing is Believing: The Power of Visualization*, Natan Sharansky, who spent nine years playing chess in his mind beat world champion chess player Garry Kasparov.[54]

The article also mentions a study by Guang Yue, an exercise psychologist from Cleveland Clinic Foundation in Ohio that compared "people who went to the gym with people who carried out virtual workouts in their heads." The study found a 30% muscle increase in the group that actually worked out. However, the group performing mental workouts also experienced a 13.5% muscle increase, which remained for 3 months.[54] This doesn't mean you can skip your exercise program - they key is to do both!

Give:

What is your passion? What would you blissfully want to spend time doing, even if you were not paid to do it? Is there a way to use that passion to bless someone else? If so, do it. Do it today.

If you're not sure, identify a single act of kindness that can bless someone else this week. Here are a few ideas:

- Leave a basket of muffins or cookies on a friend or neighbor's door.
- Invite a friend or family member over for dinner.
- Pay for a drive-thru meal or coffee for the customer behind you.
- Encourage your children to donate their slightly used toys while you donate clothes you haven't worn in the last 12 months (learn to give together).
- Surprise your husband with breakfast in bed.

Grace:

Do your Gratitude Journal each morning with prayer and Scripture reading. Be honest with God, cry out to Him with your fears, and praise Him for your blessings. Seeing His face is the midst of your worst days brings a peace that transcends our human understanding and covers the momentary circumstance with His firm and committed love. He truly comes near to the brokenhearted and has compassion for us.

Week 3:

Glow- Diet

Continue the elimination diet and remove the following additional foods: corn and refined and processed oils. Remove coffee. Make sure that your spices don't include the eliminated foods.

Add the following foods to your diet: oily cold-water and wild-caught.

Keep documenting in your Symptom Journal any increase or decrease in the frequency, type, and severity in the symptoms you experience.

Glow- Exercise:

1. Increase brisk walk or bike to 20 minutes per day
2. 3 sets of 10 abdominal crunches per day
3. 10 pushups per day
4. 50 body-weight squats 4 times a week

Gratitude:

Continue your Daily Journal and intentional action to reprogram the first toxic thought or belief. If you have the time, increase your visualization time to three minutes twice a day: morning and before bed.

Consider fasting from media news three days a week.

Give:

Continue to be a vessel of simple acts of kindness this week. Here are a few more ideas:

- Text someone a word of encouragement.
- Donate some canned goods to the local food shelter.
- Plan a time to volunteer for a local charity or your church.
- Send a thank you note to your child's teacher or your own teacher.
- Bring flowers to the office receptionist in appreciation for all he or she does.

Grace:

Continue your Gratitude Journal each morning with prayer and Bible. If you haven't downloaded the key verses from www.amongme.com/resources, do so today. The practice of writing a verse a day breathes life.

Week 4:

Glow- Diet

Maintain the elimination diet.

Keep adding to your Symptom Journal of any increase or decrease in the symptoms you experience.

Glow- Exercise:

1. Increase brisk walk or bike to 25 minutes per day
2. 3 sets of 20 abdominal crunches per day
3. 2 sets of 10 pushups per day
4. 50 body-weight squats 5 times a week

Gratitude:

You've now completed a full cycle of thought reprogramming. If you feel you still need more time reprogramming the first toxic thought or belief, then keep with the same thought for another cycle of three weeks – the work you are doing will be worth it!

If you are ready to move onto the second most toxic thought or belief, follow the same steps (see Week 1) to create a new thought or belief and intentional daily action step.

This is also a good week to create a list of your friends in whose company you feel more alive and optimistic. Be intentional to set dates to spend time with them in the coming couple of weeks.

Give:

Continue to be a vessel of simple acts of kindness this week. Here are a few more ideas:

- Talk to someone you don't know at church, school event, work function, and be intentional to just learn about their story.

- Bring a frozen meal to a friend who just had a baby, is ill, or has family who has been ill so they don't have to cook.
- Host a potluck BBQ for your neighbors.
- Bring a special coffee drink to your spouse at work.
- Write five things you love about your spouse on the bathroom mirror.

Grace:

Continue your Gratitude Journal each morning with prayer and Bible.

If you are not currently in a small group at your church, find out when enrollment starts. Be courageous and go to the group that best matches with your interest and schedule.

Week 5:

Glow- Diet

Maintain the elimination diet.

Keep adding to your Symptom Journal of any increase or decrease in the symptoms you experience.

Glow- Exercise:

1. Increase brisk walk or bike to 30 minutes per day

2. 3 sets of 20 abdominal crunches per day
3. 3 sets of 10 pushups per day
4. 50 body-weight squats 6 times a week

Gratitude:

Continue Daily Journal and intentional action to reprogram the second toxic thought or belief.

Continue the visualization exercises twice a day and fasting from media news 5 days a week.

Connect with someone who has healed from the same chronic illness you are experiencing or find a blog or book containing a similar story.

Give:

Continue to be a vessel of simple acts of kindness this week. Here are a few more ideas:
- Leave a larger tip for your server at dinner.
- Leave a note in your spouse's lunch about why you respect them.
- Listen to your son or daughter; talk about what they are most interested in for 15 minutes and ask active-listening questions.
- Plan a family game night. Get a board or card game everyone can play together. If you're single, plan a game night with some girlfriends – a themed girl night!
- Cut coupons and leave them by the items in the grocery store.

Grace:

Continue your Gratitude Journal each morning with prayer and Bible.

Week 6:

Glow- Diet

Maintain the elimination diet.

Keep adding to your Symptom Journal any increase or decrease in the symptoms you experience.

Glow- Exercise:

1. Increase brisk walk or bike to 40 minutes per day
2. 3 sets of 20 abdominal crunches; 2 sets of 25 flutter kicks per day
3. 3 sets of 10 pushups per day
4. 50 body-weight squats 7 times a week

Gratitude:

Continue Daily Journal and intentional action to reprogram the second toxic thought or belief.

Continue the visualization exercises twice a day and fasting from media news 5 days a week.

Pay attention to your dreams, especially recurring ones. Capturing what is happening in your dreams can enlighten your understanding and assist in processing your thought life.[55] Begin journaling your dreams.

Give:

Continue to be a vessel of simple acts of kindness this week. Here are a few more ideas:
- Write a card to your grandparents or have your children draw them a picture.
- Ask your mom or dad if there is an errand you could do for them today.
- Offer to do something that would normally be the role of your spouse (i.e. bath time for the kids, make dinner, dishes, etc).
- Put gas in the car of your spouse.
- Wash the car of a friend.
- Shovel snow or rake leaves for your parents, friend, or neighbor.

Grace:

Continue your Gratitude Journal each morning with prayer and Bible.

Week 7:

Glow- Diet

Oh yeah – it's time to start food reintroduction. As tempting as it is, don't rush into eating all of the eliminated foods at once. It is imperative to introduce foods one at a time and in a calculated fashion not to overwhelm your body and to properly identify the foods to which you are sensitive.

Reintroduce one of the following foods: egg yolks or legumes.

Eat one food item three times a day for two days. If you sense a reaction, stop eating that food immediately and wait until you are free of any inflammation symptoms before testing the next food. Inflammation or sensitivity to a food reaction may include the following:

- Any sign your condition is returning or worsening
- Any gastrointestinal symptoms: tummy ache, changes in bowel habits, heart burn, nausea, constipation, diarrhea, bloating
- Brian fog
- Depression
- Disruptions in sleep
- Dizziness
- Emotional
- Fatigue
- Headache
- Increased anxiety
- Joint pain or muscle aches
- Sleepiness after a meal with tested food item
- Sleeping troubles (getting or falling asleep)
- Skin changes: rashes, acne, dry skin, little pink bumps or spots, dry hair or nails
- Strong food cravings (sugar, fat, pica - mineral cravings)[56]

Once you've tested a food for two days, return to the elimination diet for three days to neutralize your system before testing the next food item.

Next foods to test (one at a time):
- Egg yolks or legumes (whichever you did not select to reintroduce in the first test).
- Seeds and nuts (not cashews or pistachios)
- Cocoa
- Chocolate
- Egg whites
- Alcohol (limited quantity)
- Eggplant
- Sweet peppers
- Paprika
- Coffee (limited quantity)
- Cashews and pistachios
- Chile peppers
- Tomatoes
- Potatoes
- White rice
- Corn (non-GMO)
- Soy (non-GMO)
- Oatmeal (gluten free)
- Quinoa
- Other gluten-free grains

Then, once you've tested each food separately for two days and returned three days back to the elimination diet, you can add back in all the foods that did not cause an inflammation or sensitivity response.

You might find that you react to a certain food earlier on in the process, but, after your gut has had some time to heal, you may be able to reintroduce that food at a later date. However, if you have a chronic condition you should eliminate gluten and cow milk dairy forever to maintain good gut health overall.[58]

You should potentially eliminate soy and corn as well due to an estimated 92% of corn and 94% of soy grown in the U.S. are genetically modified, and there has been very little research on the long-term effect of these scientifically modified foods.[59]

Amy Meyers, M.D. in her article, "3 Reasons to avoid GMO's If You Have an Autoimmune Disease," she states:

"Many GM crops, including corn, were engineered to produce their own insecticide, called Bt-toxin. Bt-toxin kills insects by destroying the lining of their digestive tracts. The poison is not specific to insects and also pokes holes in human cells, damaging the intestines and causing leaky gut, which we know is a precondition for developing an autoimmune disease."[60]

Gratitude:

You've completed the second cycle of thought or belief reprogramming. Continue to use this new skill you've developed in 3-week cycles. This is a lifelong skill and journey in neuroplasticity. Remember, your thoughts are real things with chemical reactions that bring you health or illness. Keep a filter on what thoughts you allow to take residence in your mind.

PRAYER RESOURCE

Prayer: Ask Jesus to be Your Savior & Lord

Dear God, I believe You sent Your Son Jesus to die for my sins so I can be forgiven. Forgive me for my sin and I want to live the rest of my life the way You want me to. Please put Your Spirit in my life to direct me. Amen.[62]

ABOUT BRANDIE SMITH

Brandie is an entrepreneur who founded a number of technology companies over the past twenty years. She built companies brick-by-brick from concept to generating over $100 M in retail revenue.

Some of her accomplishments include:

- Developing the Internet youth strategy for General Motors ($15 Million);
- Building what at the time was the world's largest micro-payment network worldwide by forming an alliance with over 400 carrier network operators in more than 100 countries, enabling a customer reach of over 2 billion consumers.
- Developing a patent portfolio of over 10 social networking patents for technologies being utilized today by Facebook and other social sites.

Brandie felt God calling her to leave the technology industry and spend the rest of her life serving the orphan and vulnerable child.

Supported by her husband of 9 years, Ken, and son, Zack, Brandie joined the fight to defend the fatherless for the glory of God. She now serves as the Chief Operating Officer of The Christian Alliance for Orphans (www.cafo.org).

Brandie is an active hiker, runner, and book-lover.

WORKS CITED

Chapter: Introduction

Bible: Psalm 118:17 (NIV)

Bible: Romans 12:1 (NIV)

Bible: Ephesians 4:23 (NIV)

Bible: Luke 6:31 (NIV)

Bible: Phil 4:13 (NIV)

Chapter: My Story

Bible: Joshua 1:9 (NIV)

Chapter: Information

1. The Biology Project, The University of Arizona. *Immunology Problem Set*. The University of Arizona. November 10, 2000. http://www.biology.arizona.edu/immunology/tutorials/immunology/05t.html

3. American Autoimmune Related Diseases Association, Inc. ("AARDA"). https://www.aarda.org/news-information/statistics/

4. American Autoimmune Related Diseases Association and National Coalition of Autoimmune Patient Groups. *The Cost Burden of Autoimmune Disease: The Latest Font in the War on Healthcare Spending.* 2011 http://diabetesed.net/page/_files/autoimmune-diseases.pdf

5. Mickey Trescott, NTP; Angie Alt, NTC, CHC. *The Autoimmune Wellness Handbook: A DIY Guide to living well with chronic illness.* Rodale Books (2016).

6. Amy Meyers M.D., *The Autoimmune Solution: Prevent and Reverse the Full Spectrum of Inflammatory Symptoms and Diseases.* Harper Collins Publishers (2015).

Bible. *1 Peter 5:7* (NIV)

7. Division of Nutrition, Physical Activity, and Obesity, National Center for Chronic Disease Prevention and Health Promotion. *Physical Activity and Health.* (June 2015) https://www.cdc.gov/physicalactivity/basics/pa-health/index.htm

8. LiveStrong.com. Norma Chew. *Exercise & Lymph Nodes.* August 14, 2017. https://www.livestrong.com/article/420539-exercise-lymph-nodes/

9. NCBI. US National Library of Medicine National Institutes of Health. R W Fry, J R Morton, P M Zeroni, S Gaudieri, and D Keast. *Psychological and immunological correlates of acute overtraining.* Br J Sports Med. December 1994. PMCID: PMC1332084.

10. Huffpost: Healthy Living. Leo Galland, M.D. *Do You Have Leaky Gut Syndome?.* September 2010. https://www.metsol.com/assets/sites/2/Do-you-have-leaky-gut-syndrome.pdf

Bible. *James 1:5* (NIV)

11. Dysautonomia International. *Postural Orthostatic Tachycardia Syndrome.* 2012. http://www.dysautonomiainternational.org/page.php?ID=30

12. MyHeart.Net. *POTS: Explained by Doctors & Patients.* 2151 Highland Avenue, Suite 350, Birmingham, AL 35205 https://myheart.net/pots-syndrome/pots-symptoms-signs/

Bible: *Proverbs 4:23* (NIV)

13. Dr. Caroline Leaf. *Who Switched off My Brain?* Switch on your Brain USA LLP. Published in 2009. ISBN – 10: 0-9801223-2-5. ISBN -13: 978-0-9801223-2-9.

14. MyHeart.Net. *POTS: Explained by Doctors & Patients.* 2151 Highland Avenue, Suite 350, Birmingham, AL 35205 https://myheart.net/pots-syndrome/

15. NBCI. US National Library of Medicine National Institutes of Health. Cambridge University Press. 2007. Anna Wald and Lawrence Corey. *Human Herpesviruses: Biology, Therapy, and Immunoprophylaxis. Chapter 36: Persistence in the population: epidemiology, transmission.* PMID: 21348128. https://www.ncbi.nlm.nih.gov/books/NBK47447/

16. Centers for Disease Control and Prevention: Division of STD Prevention, National Center for HIV/AIDS, Viral Hepatitis, STD, and TB Prevention, Centers for Disease Control and Prevention. *Genital Herpes – CDC Fact*

Sheet. Last updated September 1, 2017.
https://www.cdc.gov/std/herpes/stdfact-herpes.htm

17. The New York Times. Carolyn Sayre. *Students Still Getting Mono After All These Years.* January 21, 2009.
http://www.nytimes.com/ref/health/healthguide/esn-mono-ess.html

18. NCBI. US National Library of Medicine National Institutes of Health. G Vighi, F Marcucci, L Sensi, G Di Cara, and F Frati. *Allergy and the gastrointestinal system.* (Sept 2008). doi: 10.1111/j.1365-2249.2008.03713.x

19. Dr. Axe: *4 Steps to Heal Leaky Gut and Autoimmune Disease.*
https://draxe.com/4-steps-to-heal-leaky-gut-and-autoimmune-disease/

20. Dr. Axe: *7 Signs and Symptoms You Have Leaky Gut.* https://draxe.com/7-signs-symptoms-you-have-leaky-gut/

21. ChrisKresser.com. Chris Kresser. *50 Shades of Gluten.* April 23, 2013. Article featured in Huffington Post on April 3, 2013 and updated June 3, 2013. https://chriskresser.com/50-shades-of-gluten-intolerance/

Bible: *Philippians 4:8* (NIV)

Bible: *Romans 12:18* (NIV)

22. American Psychological Association. *A prospective study on volunteerism and hypertension risk in older adults.* Sneed, R.S., & Cohen, S. (2013). Psychology and Aging, 28(2), 578-586 http://psycnet.apa.org/record/2013-21685-006

23. *Romans 8:28* (NIV)

Chapter: 4 G's of Healing = Glow

Bible: *Romans 12:1* (NIV)

24. National Center for Chronic Disease Prevention and Health Promotion. *The Power of Prevention: Chronic disease...the public health challenge of the 21st century* (2009). https://www.cdc.gov/chronicdisease/pdf/2009-power-of-prevention.pdf

25. Michael Finkelstein, M.D. *Slow Medicine: Hope and Healing for Chronic Illness.* HaperCollins Publishers (2013). ISBN 978-0-06-222552-8.

26. Angela M. Zivkovic, Natalie Telis, J. Bruce German, and Bruce D. Hammock. *Dietary omega-3 fatty acids in the modulation of inflammation and metabolic health.* Published on PMC: US National Library of medicine National Institues of Health. Published in final edited form as: Calif Agric (Berkeley). 2011 July-September; 65(3): 106–111. doi: 10.3733/ca.v065n03p106

27. Dr. Josh Axe, DNM, DC, CNS. *4 Steps to Heal Leaky Gut and Autoimmune Disease.* https://draxe.com/4-steps-to-heal-leaky-gut-and-autoimmune-disease/

2. Dr. Mercola. https://articles.mercola.com/sites/articles/archive/2008/07/05/probiotics-found-to-help-your-gut-s-immune-system.aspx

28. Dr. Josh Axe, DNM, DC, CNS. *Vitamin K Deficiency, Foods & Health Benefits.* https://draxe.com/vitamin-k-deficiency/

1. The Biology Project, The University of Arizona. *Immunology Problem Set.* The University of Arizona. November 10, 2000. http://www.biology.arizona.edu/immunology/tutorials/immunology/05t.html.

29. Dr. Jill. Carnahan. https://www.jillcarnahan.com/2014/07/07/leaky-gut-syndrome-linked-many-autoimmune-diseases/.

31. ChrisKresser.com. Chris Kresser. *50 Shades of Gluten.* April 23, 2013. Article featured in Huffington Post on April 3, 2013 and updated June 3, 2013. https://chriskresser.com/50-shades-of-gluten-intolerance/

32. Sarah Ballantyne, PhD. https://www.thepaleomom.com/

33. Amy Meyers, M.D. *The Autoimmune Solution: Food Reintroduction Bonus:* https://www.amymyersmd.com/wp-content/uploads/2015/08/BonusMaterial.pdf

34. Dr. James DiNicolantonio. *The Salt Fix: Why the Experts Got it All Wrong – and How Eating More Might Save Your Life.* Harmony 2017. ISBN: 978-0-451-49696-6.

35. MyHeart.Net. POTS: *Explained by Doctors & Patients.* 2151 Highland Avenue, Suite 350, Birmingham, AL 35205 https://myheart.net/pots-syndrome/

36. Sarah Ballantyne, PhD. https://www.thepaleomom.com/start-here/the-autoimmune-protocol/

37. Division of Nutrition, Physical Activity, and Obesity, National Center for Chronic Disease Prevention and Health Promotion. *Physical Activity and Health.* (June 2015) https://www.cdc.gov/physicalactivity/basics/pa-health/index.htm

38. Heathline. *The Top 10 Benefits of Regular Exercise.* Authority Nutrition. https://www.healthline.com/nutrition/10-benefits-of-exercise#section4

Chapter: 4 G's of Healing = Gratitude

Bible: *Philippians 4:6* (NIV)

39. Michael Finkelstein, M.D. *Slow Medicine: Hope and Healing for Chronic Illness.* HaperCollins Publishers (2013). ISBN 978-0-06-222552-8.

40. Dr. Carloine Leaf. Toxic Thoughts. http://drleaf.com/about/toxic-thoughts/

Bible: *Matthew 18: 24-25* (NIV)

Bible: *Philippians 4:13* (NIV)

Bible: *Psalm 118:17* (NIV)

Bible: *Exodus 14:14* (NIV)

Bible: *Philippians 4:8* (NIV)

Bible: *2 Timothy 1:7* (NIV)

Bible: *Philippians 4:7* (NIV)

Bible: *Philippians 4:6* (NIV)

Bible: *1 Peter 5:7* (NIV)

Bible: *Psalm 46:1* (NIV)

Bible: *Philippians 3:13-14* (NIV)

42. Karen Swartz. John Hopkins article: *Forgiveness: Your Health Depends on It.* http://www.hopkinsmedicine.org/health/healthy_aging/healthy_connectio ns/forgiveness-your-health-depends-on-it

43. John Hopkins article: *Forgiveness: Your Health Depends on It.* http://www.hopkinsmedicine.org/health/healthy_aging/healthy_connectio ns/forgiveness-your-health-depends-on-it

Bible: *Romans 12:18* (NIV).

44. Benjamin Franklin quote: He that has once done you a kindness will be more ready to do you another, than he whom you yourself have obliged.

Forbes. Jonathan Becher, SAP. *Do Me a Favor So You'll Like Me: The Reverse Psychology of Likeability.* November 16, 2011.
https://www.forbes.com/sites/sap/2011/11/16/do-me-a-favor-so-youll-like-me-the-reverse-psychology-of-likeability/#1651c60c74a5

Bible: *Psalm 118:24* (NIV)

Chapter: 4 G's of Healing = Give

Bible: *Proverbs 11:25* (NIV)

Bible: *Philippians 4:13* (NIV)

45. Hilary Young. Huffingtonpost.com article, *Why Volunteering Is So Good For Your Health.* November 1, 2013. Article cites study by UnitedHealth Group. https://www.huffingtonpost.com/hilary-young/benefits-of-volunteering_b_4151540.html

Chapter: 4 G's of Healing = Grace

Bible: *Philippians 4:4* (NIV)
46. Huffpost. Don Joseph Goeway. *85 Percent of What We Worry About Never Happens.* Aug 2015; updated Dec 2017.
https://www.huffingtonpost.com/don-joseph-goewey-/85-of-what-we-worry-about_b_8028368.html

Bible: *Matthew 6:27* (NIV)

Bible: *Matthew 6:34* (NIV)

Bible: *Philippians 4:6-7* (NIV)

Bible: *Philippians 4:8* (NIV)

Bible: *Ecclesiastes 4:6* (GN)

Chapter: 6-Week 4 G's of Healing Plan

47. Dr. Andrew Weil, M.D. *8 Weeks to Optimal Health: A Proven Program for Taking Full Advantage of Your Body's Natural Healing Power.* Ballantine Books, an imprint of the Random House Publishing Group, a Division of Random House, Inc., New York. 2006. ISBN: 978-0-345-49802-1

Mickey Trescott, NTP; Angie Alt, NTC, CHC.
http://autoimmunewellness.com/recipes/

Amy Meyers M.D., https://www.amymyersmd.com/recipes/

48. National Institute of Neurological Disorders and Stroke, National Institutes of Health. *Brain Basics: Understanding Sleep.* Bethesda, MD 20892. NIH Publication No. 17-3440-c

49. NCBI. US National Library of Medicine National Institutes of Health. Kelly Glazor Baron, PdD, MPH and Katheryn J. Reid PhD. *Circadian Misalignment and Health.* PMC 2015 Dec 14. doi: 10.3109/09540261.2014.911149.
https://www.ncbi.nlm.nih.gov/pmc/articles/PMC4677771/

50. Dr. Caroline Leaf. *Who Switched off My Brain?* Switch on your Brain USA LLP. Published in 2009. ISBN – 10: 0-9801223-2-5. ISBN -13: 978-0-9801223-2-9.

51. Huffpost. Debbie Hampton. *How Your Thoughts Change Your Brain, Cells and Genes.* March 23, 2016 and updated March 24, 2017. https://www.huffingtonpost.com/debbie-hampton/how-your-thoughts-change-your-brain-cells-and-genes_b_9516176.html

52. Carnegie Mellon University: Open Learning Initiative. Introduction to Psychology. Module 5: Neurotransmitters: The Body's Chemical Messengers. https://oli.cmu.edu/jcourse/workbook/activity/page?context=434a8f9e800 20ca6012e0a70c3d80523

53. Sarah Ballantyne, PhD. https://www.thepaleomom.com/start-here/the-autoimmune-protocol/

54. AJ Adams, MAPP. *Seeing is Believing: The Power of Visualization.* Psychology Today. December 3, 2009. https://www.psychologytoday.com/blog/flourish/200912/seeing-is-believing-the-power-visualization

55. KPBS: Nova. Robert Stickgold. *Dreams: Expert Q& A.* November 30,2009. http://www.pbs.org/wgbh/nova/body/stickgold-dreams.html

56. Sarah Ballantyne, PhD. https://www.thepaleomom.com/reintroducing-foods-after-following-the-autoimmune-protocol/

58. Amy Meyers, M.D. *The Autoimmune Solution: Food Reintroduction Bonus*: https://www.amymyersmd.com/wp-content/uploads/2015/08/BonusMaterial.pdf

59. United States Department of Agriculture: Economic Research Service. *Recent Trends in GE Adooption*. July 12, 2017. https://www.ers.usda.gov/data-products/adoption-of-genetically-engineered-crops-in-the-us/recent-trends-in-ge-adoption.aspx

60. Amy Meyers, M.D. *3 Reasons to Avoid GMOs If You Have an Autoimmune Disease*. https://www.amymyersmd.com/2017/08/3-reasons-to-avoid-gmos-if-you-have-an-autoimmune-disease/

61. Harvard Health Publishing, Harvard Medical School. *Anxiety and physical illness: Understanding and treating anxiety can often improve the outcome of chronic disease*. Published July 2008 and updated June 6, 2017. https://www.health.harvard.edu/staying-healthy/anxiety_and_physical_illness

62. Coastline Church. 2215 Calle Barcelona, Carlsbad, CA 92009 http://www.coastlinechurch.org